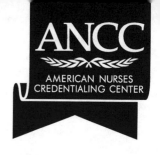

NURSING REVIEW AND RESOURCE MANUAL

Nursing Professional Development

Published by American Nurses Credentialing Center
Authors: Diane D. DePew, DSN, RN-BC, and Patricia Kummeth, MSN, RN-BC

CONTINUING EDUCATION SOURCE
NURSING CERTIFICATION REVIEW MANUAL
CLINICAL PRACTICE RESOURCE

2nd Edition

Library of Congress Cataloging-in-Publication Data

DePew, Diane.
  Nursing professional development review and resource manual. – 2nd ed. / Diane DePew and Patricia Kummeth.
       p. ; cm.
  Rev. ed. of: Nursing professional development review and resource manual / Adrianne Avillion, Barbara Brunt, Mary Jane Ferrell. c2007.
  Includes bibliographical references and index.
  ISBN 978-1-935213-19-2 (alk. paper)
  1. Nurses–In-service training–United States–Handbooks, manuals, etc. I. Kummeth, Patricia. II. Avillion, Adrianne E. Nursing professional development review and resource manual . III. American Nurses Credentialing Center. IV. Title.
  [DNLM: 1. Education, Nursing, Continuing–Outlines. 2. Nursing Staff–education–Outlines. 3. Staff Development–methods–Outlines. 4. Teaching–methods–Outlines. WY 18.2]
  RT76.A95 2011
  610.73071'5–dc22
                          2010053688

The American Nurses Credentialing Center (ANCC), a subsidiary of the American Nurses Association (ANA), provides individuals and organizations throughout the nursing profession with the resources they need to achieve practice excellence. ANCC's internationally renowned credentialing programs certify nurses in specialty practice areas; recognize healthcare organizations for promoting safe, positive work environments through the Magnet Recognition Program® and the Pathway to Excellence ® Program; and accredit providers of continuing nursing education. In addition, ANCC's Institute for Credentialing Innovation provides leading-edge information and education services and products to support its core credentialing programs.

ISBN 13: 978-1-935213-19-2
© 2011 American Nurses Credentialing Center.
8515 Georgia Ave., Suite 400
Silver Spring, MD 20910

Nursing Professional Development Review and Resource Manual, 2nd Edition

FEBRUARY 2011

Please direct your comments and/or queries to: revmanuals@ana.org

The healthcare services delivery system is a volatile marketplace demanding superior knowledge, clinical skills, and competencies from all registered nurses. Nursing autonomy of practice and nurse career marketability and mobility in the new century hinge on affirming the profession's formative philosophy, which places a priority on a lifelong commitment to the principles of education and professional development. The knowledge base of nursing theory and practice is expanding, and while care has been taken to ensure the accuracy and timeliness of the information presented in the **Nursing Professional Development Review and Resource Manual, 2nd Edition**, clinicians are advised to always verify the most current national guidelines and recommendations and to practice in accordance with professional standards of care used with regard to the unique circumstances that apply in each practice situation. In addition, the editors wish to note that provision of information in this text does not imply an endorsement of any particular products, procedures or services.

Therefore, the authors, editors, American Nurses Association (ANA), American Nurses Association's Publishing (ANP), American Nurses Credentialing Center (ANCC), and the Institute for Credentialing Innovation cannot accept responsibility for errors or omissions, or for any consequences or liability, injury, and/or damages to persons or property from application of the information in this manual and make no warranty, express or implied, with respect to the contents of the **Nursing Professional Development Review and Resource Manual, 2nd Edition**. Completion of this manual does not guarantee that the reader will pass the certification exam.

Published by:
American Nurses Credentialing Center
The Institute for Credentialing Innovation
8515 Georgia Avenue, Suite 400
Silver Spring, MD 20910-3402
www.nursecredentialing.org

Introduction to the Continuing Education (CE) Contact Hour Application Process for *Nursing Professional Development Review and Resource Manual, 2nd Edition*

The Institute for Credentialing Innovation now offers the continuing education contact hours for this manual online at www.NursingWorld.org, the American Nurses Association's Web site. This process involves answering approximately 25–30 questions that test knowledge of the information contained within this manual. The continuing education contact hours can be completed at any time and a certificate can be printed from the Web site immediately upon successful completion of the test.

After studying the manual and given an online multiple-choice test, the exam candidate will be able to:

1. Pass the posttest with at least 75% of the answers correct.
2. Select responses to test questions based on key principles, standards of practice, and theoretical basis of nursing practice.
3. Choose accepted therapeutic interventions in answering questions related to quality nursing practice.
4. Utilize direct and indirect professional role responsibilities and applications regarding nursing practice in answering test questions.

Upon completion of this manual and the online CE test, a nurse can receive a total of 15 continuing education contact hours at a price of $30, only $2 per CE. (ANA members receive a discount on CEs.) **The entire process—online test and evaluation form—must be completed by December 31, 2013 in order to receive credit.** To begin the process, please e-mail **revmanuals@ana.org**. Your patience with this process is greatly appreciated.

Inquiries or Comments

If you have any questions about the CE contact hours, please e-mail The Institute at revmanuals@ana.org. You may also mail any comments to Editor/Project Manager, at the address listed below.

Duplicate CE Certificates

Once you have successfully passed the CE test, you may go back and re-print your certificate as often as you wish.

Conflicts of Interest

A conflict of interest occurs when an individual has an opportunity to affect educational content about health-care products or services of a commercial company with which she/he has a financial relationship.

The planners and presenters of this CNE activity have disclosed no relevant financial relationships with any commercial companies pertaining to this activity.

The Institute for Credentialing Innovation
American Nurses Credentialing Center
Attn: Editor/Project Manager
8515 Georgia Avenue, Suite 400
Silver Spring, MD 20910-3492
Fax: (301) 628-5342

A maximum of 15 contact hours may be earned by learners who successfully complete this continuing nursing education activity.

The American Nurses Association Center for Continuing Education and Professional Development is accredited as a provider of continuing nursing education by the American Nurses Credentialing Center's Commission on Accreditation.

ANCC Provider Number 0023

ANA is approved by the California Board of Registered Nursing, Provider Number 6178.

The ANA Center for Continuing Education and Professional Development includes ANCC's Institute for Credentialing Innovation.

Acknowledgements

The editors gratefully acknowledge the foundational work provided by the authors of the previous edition:

Adrianne Avillion, DEd, RN
Barbara Brunt, MA, MN, RN-BC
Mary Jane Ferrell, PhD, RN-BC

NOTE ABOUT THE *NURSING PROFESSIONAL DEVELOPMENT SCOPE & STANDARDS OF PRACTICE*

The ANCC *Nursing Professional Development Review and Resource Manual, 2nd edition* was written to help nurses prepare for the ANCC Nursing Professional Development Certification exam that is based on the test content outline effective November 1, 2008. This current exam, which will be used through early 2012, incorporates the *Nursing Professional Development Scope and Standards of Practice* from 2000. Because these are the standards included on the exam, we have used those standards in the text.

The new standards, released in 2010, will be used for the 2012 exam; at that time, this text will be revised to incorporate them.

Contents

NURSING PROFESSIONAL DEVELOPMENT REVIEW AND RESOURCE MANUAL

2ND EDITION

Taking the Certification Examination

When you sign up to take a national certification exam, you will be instructed to go online and review the testing and review handbook (www.nursecredentialing.org/documents/certification/ application/generaltestingandrenewalhandbook.aspx). Review it carefully and be sure to bookmark the site so you can refer to it frequently. It contains information on test content and sample questions. This is critical information; it will give you insight into the nature of the test. The agency will send you information about the test site; keep this in a safe place until needed.

GENERAL SUGGESTIONS FOR PREPARING FOR THE EXAM

Step One: Control Your Anxiety

Everyone experiences anxiety when faced with taking the certification exam.

- Remember, your program was designed to prepare you to take this exam.
- Your instructors took a similar exam, and have probably talked to students who took exams more recently, so they know how to help you prepare.
- Taking a review course or setting up your own study plan will help you feel more confident about taking the exam.

Step Two: Do Not Listen to Gossip About the Exam

A large volume of information exists about the tests based on reports from people who have taken the exams in the past. Because information from the testing facilities is limited, it is hard to ignore this gossip.

- Remember that gossip about the exam that you hear from others is not verifiable.
- Because this gossip is based on the imperfect memory of people in a stressful situation, it may not be very accurate.
- People tend to remember those items testing content with which they are less comfortable; for instance, those with a limited background in women's health may say that the exam was "all women's health." In fact, the exam blueprint ensures that the exam covers multiple content areas without overemphasizing any one.

Step Three: Set Reasonable Expectations for Yourself

- Do not expect to know everything.
- Do not try to know everything in great detail.
- You do not need a perfect score to pass the exam.
- The exam is designed for a beginner level—it is testing readiness for entry-level practice.
- Learn the general rules, not the exceptions.
- The most likely diagnoses will be on the exam, not questions on rare diseases or atypical cases.
- Think about the most likely presentation and most common therapy.

Step Four: Prepare Mentally and Physically

- While you are getting ready to take the exam, take good physical care of yourself.
- Get plenty of sleep and exercise, and eat well while preparing for the exam.
- These things are especially important while you are studying and immediately before you take the exam.

Step Five: Access Current Knowledge

General Content
You will be given a list of general topics that will be on the exam when you register to take the exam. In addition, examine the table of contents of this book and the test content outline, available at www.nursecredentialing.org/cert/TCOs.html.
- What content do you need to know?
- How well do you know these subjects?

Take a Review Course
- Taking a review course is an excellent way to assess your knowledge of the content that will be included in the exam.
- If you plan to take a review course, take it well before the exam so you will have plenty of time to master any areas of weakness the course uncovers.

- If you are prepared for the exam, you will not hear anything new in the course. You will be familiar with everything that is taught.
- If some topics in the review course are new to you, concentrate on these in your studies.
- People have a tendency to study what they know; it is rewarding to study something and feel a mastery of it! Unfortunately, this will not help you master unfamiliar content. Be sure to use a review course to identify your areas of strength and weakness, then concentrate on the weaknesses.

Depth of Knowledge

How much do you need to know about a subject?
- You cannot know everything about a topic.
- Remember that the depth of knowledge required to pass the exam is for entry-level performance.
- Study the information sent to you from the testing agency, what you were taught in school, what is covered in this text, and the general guidelines given in this chapter.
- Look at practice tests designed for the exam. Practice tests for other exams will not be helpful.
- Consult your class notes or clinical diagnosis and management textbook for the major points about a disease. Additional reference books can be found online at www.nursecredentialing.org/cert/refs.html.
- For example, with regard to medications, know the drug categories and the major medications in each. Assume all drugs in a category are generally alike, and then focus on the differences among common drugs. Know the most important indications, contraindications, and side effects. Emphasize safety. The questions usually do not require you to know the exact dosage of a drug.

Step Six: Institute a Systematic Study Plan

Develop Your Study Plan
- Write a formal plan of study.
  - Include topics for study, timetable, resources, and methods of study that work for you.
  - Decide whether you want to organize a study group or work alone.
  - Schedule regular times to study.
  - Avoid cramming; it is counterproductive. Try to schedule your study periods in 1-hour increments.
- Identify resources to use for studying. To prepare for the examination, you should have the following materials on your shelf:
  - A good pathophysiology text.
  - This review book.
  - A physical assessment text.
  - Your class notes.
  - Other important sources, including: information from the testing facility, a clinical diagnosis textbook, favorite journal articles, notes from a review course, and practice tests.
  - Know the important national standards of care for major illnesses.

– Consult the bibliography on the test blueprint. When studying less familiar material, it is helpful to study using the same references that the testing center uses.
– Study the body systems from head to toe.
– The exams emphasize health promotion, assessment, differential diagnosis, and plan of care for common problems.
– You will need to know facts and be able to interpret and analyze this information utilizing critical thinking.

Personalize Your Study Plan
• How do you learn best?
   – If you learn best by listening or talking, attend a review course or discuss topics with a colleague.
• Read everything the test facility sends you as soon as you receive it and several times during your preparation period. It will give you valuable information to help guide your study.
• Have a specific place with good lighting set aside for studying. Find a quiet place with no distractions. Assemble your study materials.

Implement Your Study Plan
You must have basic content knowledge. In addition, you must be able to use this information to think critically and make decisions based on facts.
• Refer to your study plan regularly.
• Stick to your schedule.
• Take breaks when you get tired.
• If you start procrastinating, get help from a friend or reorganize your study plan.
• It is not necessary to follow your plan rigidly. Adjust as you learn where you need to spend more time.
• Memorize the basics of the content areas you will be required to know.

Focus on General Material
• Most of what you need to know is basic material that does not require constant updating.
• You do not need to worry about the latest information being published as you are studying for the exam. Remember, it can take 6 to 12 months for new information to be incorporated into test questions.

Pace Your Studying
• Stop studying for the examination when you are starting to feel overwhelmed and look at what is bothering you. Then make changes.
• Break overwhelming tasks into smaller tasks that you know you can do.
• Stop and take breaks while studying.

Work With Others
• Talk with classmates about your preparation for the exam.
• Keep in touch with classmates, and help each other stick to your study plans.
• If your classmates become anxious, do not let their anxiety affect you. Walk away if you need to.
• Do not believe bad stories you hear about other people's experiences with previous exams.
• Remember, you know as much as anyone about what will be on the next exam!

Consider a Study Group
- Study groups can provide practice in analyzing cases, interpreting questions, and critical thinking.
  - You can discuss a topic and take turns presenting cases for the group to analyze.
  - Study groups also can provide moral support and help you continue studying.

Step Seven: Strategies Immediately Before the Exam

Final Preparation Suggestions
- Use practice exams when studying to get accustomed to the exam format and time restrictions.
  - Many books that are labeled as review books are simply a collection of examination questions.
  - If you have test anxiety, such practice tests may help alleviate the anxiety.
  - Practice tests can help you learn to judge the time it should take you to complete the exam.
  - Practice tests are useful for gaining experience in analyzing questions.
  - Books of questions may not uncover the gaps in your knowledge that a more systematic content review text will reveal.
  - If you feel that you don't know enough about a topic, refer to a text to learn more. After you feel that you have learned the topic, practice questions are a wonderful tool to help improve your test-taking skill.
- Know your test-taking style.
  - Do you rush through the exam without reading the questions thoroughly?
  - Do you get stuck and dwell on a question for a long time?
  - You should spend about 45 to 60 seconds per question and finish with time to review the questions you were not sure about.
  - Be sure to read the question completely, including all four answer choices. Choice "a" may be good, but "d" may be best.

The Night Before the Exam
- Be prepared to get to the exam on time.
  - Know the test site location and how long it takes to get there.
  - Take a "dry run" beforehand to make sure you know how to get to the testing site, if necessary.
  - Get a good night's sleep.
  - Eat sensibly.
  - Avoid alcohol the night before.
- Assemble the required material—two forms of identification, admission card, pencil, and watch. Both IDs must match the name on the application, and one photo ID is preferred.
- Know the exam room rules.
  - You will be given scratch paper, which will be collected at the end of the exam.
  - Nothing else is allowed in the exam room.
  - You will be required to put papers, backpacks, etc., in a corner of the room or in a locker.
  - No water or food will be allowed.
  - You will be allowed to walk to a water fountain and go to the bathroom one at a time.

The Day of the Exam
- Get there early. If you are late, you may not be admitted.
- Think positively. You have studied hard and are well-prepared.
- Remember your anxiety reduction strategies.

Specific Tips for Dealing With Anxiety

Test anxiety is a specific type of anxiety. Symptoms include upset stomach, sweaty palms, tachycardia, trouble concentrating, and a feeling of dread. But there are ways to cope with test anxiety.

- There is no substitute for being well-prepared.
- Practice relaxation techniques.
- Avoid alcohol, excess coffee, caffeine, and any new medications that might sedate you, dull your senses, or make you feel agitated.
- Take a few deep breaths and concentrate on the task at hand.

Focus on Specific Test-Taking Skills

To do well on the exam, you need good test-taking skills in addition to knowledge of the content and ability to use critical thinking.

All Certification Exams Are Multiple Choice

- Multiple-choice tests have specific rules for test construction.
- A multiple-choice question consists of three parts: the information (or stem), the question, and the four possible answers (one correct and three distracters).
- Careful analysis of each part is necessary. Read the entire question before answering.
- Practice your test-taking skills by analyzing the practice questions in this book and on the ANCC Web site.

Analyze the Information Given

- Do not assume you have more information than is given.
- Do not overanalyze.
- Remember, the writer of the question assumes this is all of the information needed to answer the question.
- If information is not given, it is not relevant and will not affect the answer.
- Do not make the question more complicated than it is.

What Kind of Question Is Asked?

- Are you supposed to recall a fact, apply facts to a situation, or understand and differentiate between options?

- Read the question thinking about what the writer is asking.
- Look for key words or phrases that lead you (see Figure 1–1). These help determine what kind of answer the question requires.

Figure 1–1. Examples of Key Words and Phrases

- avoid
- best
- except
- not
- initial

- first
- contributing to
- appropriate
- most
- significant

- likely
- of the following
- most consistent with

Read All of the Answers

- If you are absolutely certain that answer "a" is correct as you read it, mark it, but read the rest of the question so you do not trick yourself into missing a better answer.
- If you are absolutely sure answer "a" is wrong, cross it off or make a note on your scratch paper and continue reading the question.
- After reading the entire question, go back, analyze the question, and select the best answer.
- Do not jump ahead.
- If the question asks you for an assessment, the best answer will be an assessment. Do not be distracted by an intervention that sounds appropriate.
- If the question asks you for an intervention, do not answer with an assessment.
- When two answer choices sound very good, the best one is usually the least expensive, least invasive way to achieve the goal. For example, if your answer choices include a physical exam maneuver or imaging, the physical exam maneuver is probably the better choice provided it will give the information needed.
- If the answers include two options that are the opposite of each other, one of the two is probably the correct answer.
- When numeric answers cover a wide range, a number in the middle is more likely to be correct.
- Watch out for distracters that are correct but do not answer the question, combine true and false information, or contain a word or phrase that is similar to the correct answer.
- Err on the side of caution.

Only One Answer Can Be Correct

- When more than one suggested answer is correct, you must identify the one that best answers the question asked.
- If you cannot choose between two answers, you have a 50% chance of getting it right if you guess.

Avoid Changing Answers

- Change an answer only if you have a compelling reason, such as you remembered something additional, or you understand the question better after rereading it.
- People change to a wrong answer more often than to a right answer.

Time Yourself to Complete the Whole Exam

- Do not spend a large amount of time on one question.
- If you cannot answer a question quickly, mark it and continue the exam.
- If time is left at the end, return to the difficult questions.
- Make educated guesses by eliminating the obviously wrong answers and choosing a likely answer even if you are not certain.
- Trust your instinct.
- Answer every question. There is no penalty for a wrong answer.
- Occasionally a question will remind you of something that helps you with a question earlier in the test. Look back at that question to see if what you are remembering affects how you would answer that question.

ABOUT THE CERTIFICATION EXAMS

The American Nurses Credentialing Center Computerized Exam

The ANCC examination is given only as a computer exam, and each exam is different. The order of the questions is scrambled for every test, so even if two people are taking the same exam, the questions will be in a different order. The exam consists of 175 multiple-choice questions.

- 150 of the 175 questions are part of the test and how you answer will count toward your score; 25 are included to refine questions and will not be scored. You will not know which ones count, so treat all questions the same.
- You will need to know how to use a mouse, scroll by either clicking arrows on the scroll bar or using the up and down arrow keys, and perform other basic computer tasks.
- The exam does not require computer expertise.
- However, if you are not comfortable with using a computer, you should practice using a mouse and computer beforehand so you do not waste time on the mechanics of using the computer.

Know what to expect during the test.
- Each ANCC test question is independent of the other questions.
  - For each case study, there is only one question. This means that a correct answer on any question does not depend on the correct answer to any other question.
  - Each question has four possible answers. There are no questions asking for combinations of correct answers (such as "a and c") or multiple-multiples.

- You can skip a question and go back to it at the end of the exam.
- You cannot mark key words in the question or right or wrong answers. If you want to do this, use the scratch paper.
- You will get your results immediately, and a grade report will be provided upon leaving the testing site.

INTERNET RESOURCES

- ANCC Web site: www.nursecredentialing.org
- ANA Bookstore: www.nursesbooks.org. Catalog of ANA nursing scope and standards publications and other titles that may be listed on your test content outline
- National Guideline Clearinghouse: www.ngc.gov

2

Organizational Factors

DEFINITIONS

- *Culture* refers to the personality of an organization that is determined by various *dynamics* present in the workplace (Andrews & Boyle, 2008).
- *Dynamics* are defined as the interacting forces within a group that produce a pattern or process of change, growth, or activity (Merriam-Webster, 2010).
- The *purpose* is the reason for the existence of an organization or department.
- The words *purpose* and *mission* often are used interchangeably.
- A *mission statement* is a statement of purpose that defines the direction and target of an organization's activities.
- A *vision* is a statement that describes the desired future of an organization or a department.
- *Values* are beliefs and principles that describe the way an organization directs its activities (Abruzzese, 1996).
- *Goals* are broad statements that describe the object or end that one strives to attain (ANCC, 2009).

ORGANIZATIONAL CULTURE AND DYNAMICS

- The vision, mission, values, assumptions, norms, and other factors that influence the dynamics in an organization determine the organizational culture.

- Organizational dynamics integrate the analytical work of an organization with the emotional processes of its people. It is influenced by leadership and management styles, number of employees, and geographic locations.
- Informal factors such as assumptions and historical norms also may influence the organizational dynamics and hence, the culture within an organization. For example, individuals may maintain and expect behavior that is consistent with well-established traditions about teamwork expectations, meeting behavior, or dress code.
- The organizational culture establishes patterns for individuals to understand particular events, actions, communications, or situations within the organization. These patterns of understanding help individuals manage their behavior as they encounter new experiences in the work environment.
- In addition, demographic factors such as size, location, geographic setting, and number of employees also contribute to the organizational culture (Andrews & Boyle, 2008).
- Examples of healthcare organizations with distinctly different cultures include:
  - 50-bed rural critical access hospital
  - 800-bed tertiary care center in a metropolitan area
  - 500-bed hospital affiliated with a university
  - 45-bed long-term care and hospice facility
  - 200-bed military hospital and clinic

MISSION

- The mission describes essential functions of an organization or department as well as the reason for its existence (Avillion, 2008).
  - Mission statements clearly and concisely communicate the purpose and direction of an entity's activities.
  - Vision is an image or dream of the desired future of an organization.
  - Values (sometimes referred to as philosophy) are beliefs and principles that direct an organization's activities.
- A mission statement identifies the composition and scope of the department or organization, the reason for existence, and the target audience being served.
- The mission statement provides clear direction toward achieving established goals and objectives and an explicit definition to employees (Abruzzese, 1996).
- The mission statement for an education department or program is developed using the organization's mission statement. The departmental mission must reflect the values and beliefs of the department and the organization (Penn, 2008).
- A well-written mission statement for a nursing professional development department reflects the organizational mission, values, and vision; focuses on organizational and departmental priorities; serves as the foundation for departmental goals and objectives; and evolves and changes as the organization's priorities change (Avillion, 2008).

- Sample mission statement: The staff development department of General Healthcare System supports the mission, vision, and values of the organization by developing and providing educational products and services designed to enhance the quality of patient care. This is accomplished through educational activities intended to increase knowledge and skills of employees in the nursing division. The department is committed to conducting and analyzing research data to identify benchmarks and best practices in the field of nursing professional development.

VISION

- A clear and attainable vision creates value. It is inspiring and exciting for employees as they strive individually and collaboratively to achieve the identified future state.
- A vision, as the ideal image of a desired state, provides everyone involved with a common identity and sense of purpose (Abruzzese, 1996).
- A vision must be precise, realistic, easily understood, and clearly written so that it is meaningful to both employees, patients, and stakeholders (Avillion, 2008).
- Sample vision statement: It is the vision of the education and professional development division to be a regional leader in the provision of education programs that focus on excellence in oncology healthcare services and to conduct educational research for the purpose of identifying best practices in continuing education for oncology nurses.

VALUES

- The values and beliefs of a department or organization are expressed in the philosophy.
- Values serve as the foundational principles that guide all the actions of a department or organization (Kelly-Thomas, 1998).
- Values may be incorporated into mission statements or may supplement a mission statement as a declaration of what is important to the department (Golway, 2009).
- Values exert a powerful influence on how each individual chooses to react and behave in specific situations (Andrews & Boyle, 2008).
- For employees of a department to live its values, the following must occur:
  - Employees use the established values to guide their work performance, priority-setting, decision-making, and interactions.
  - Rewards and recognition are awarded to individuals whose work reflects the departmental values.
  - Recruitment and retention efforts focus on hiring and keeping persons whose work behaviors are congruent with the departmental values (Heathfield, 2007).
- Factors that affect nursing professional development may influence the values of an educational department or organization. These factors include:
  - Environment: patient population, demographics, healthcare delivery systems, cultural variations in staff and patient groups, setting
  - Learner characteristics: learning style, educational background, experience, personal values
  - Educational design: classroom, online, independent study, audio or teleconference (Kelly-Thomas, 1998)

- Consistent values across all levels of an organization result in fewer conflicts and greater commitment by all employees.
- Values that guided the development of the scope and standards for nursing professional development incorporate the following concepts (ANA, 2000):
  - Lifelong learning
  - Professional nursing competence
  - Roles of the nursing professional development educator
  - Self-directed, active learner role
  - Adult learning principles
  - Educational options
  - Evaluation

GOALS

- Goals are broadly written statements that guide an organization to complete activities that will contribute to achievement of the mission.
- Goals for a nursing professional development department must be based on relevant, appropriate organizational goals so that educational efforts contribute to achievement of the organization's goals (Avillion, 2008).
- Although goals are derived from the mission and values of the department, they are more concrete and specific to serve as a basis for developing more detailed outcomes for specific programmatic areas.
- Because the primary mission of nursing professional development is to provide educational programs and services, departmental goal statements cover programmatic areas such as orientation, continuing education, competency assessment, and in-service.
- Goals may focus on the outcomes of programmatic areas in education or on the educational processes used to achieve these outcomes (Kelly-Thomas, 1998).
- Goals in the educational process are broad, global statements of the final outcomes to be achieved at the end of the teaching and learning processes.
- Educational goals are multidimensional; they incorporate several specific objectives of a learning activity (Bastable, 2008).
- The goals of a nursing professional development department change as the needs and priorities of the organization change.
- Because goals of a nursing professional development department evolve as the organization evolves, it is important to conduct a periodic, systematic review to confirm, revise, or update the goals to ensure that they remain consistent with the direction of the organization (Alspach, 1995).
- Sample goals for a nursing professional development department:
  - By the end of the fiscal year, 50% of the rehabilitation staff nurses will complete a certification review course in their clinical specialty.
  - Use of the simulation center for emergency response training updates will be implemented in all critical care areas within the next six months.
  - The nursing professional development department will reduce printing expenditures by 10% through conversion to electronic communication and documentation.

REFERENCES

Abruzzese, R. S. (Ed.). (1996). *Nursing staff development: Strategies for success.* St. Louis, MO: Mosby.

Alspach, J. G. (1995). *The educational process in nursing staff development.* St. Louis, MO: Mosby.

American Nurses Association. (2000). *Scope and standards of practice for nursing professional development.* Silver Spring, MD: American Nurses Publishing.

American Nurses Credentialing Center's Commission on Accreditation. (2009). *Application manual: Accreditation program.* Silver Spring, MD: American Nurses Credentialing Center.

Andrews, M. M., & Boyle, J. S. (2008). *Transcultural concepts in nursing care* (5th ed.). Philadelphia: Lippincott Williams & Wilkins.

Avillion, A. E. (2008). *A practical guide to staff development: Evidence-based tools and techniques for effective education* (2nd ed.). Marblehead, MA: HCPro.

Bastable, S. B. (2008). *Nurse as educator: Principles of teaching and learning for nursing practice.* Boston: Jones & Bartlett.

Dynamics. (2010). *Merriam-Webster Online Dictionary.* Retrieved from http://www.merriam-webster.com/dictionary/dynamics

Golway, M. M. (2009). Purpose, philosophy, and objectives. In S. L. Bruce (Ed.), *Core curriculum for staff development* (3rd ed., pp. 21-32). Pensacola, PA: National Nursing Staff Development Organization.

Heathfield, S. (2007). *Build a strategic framework: Mission statement, vision, values.* About.com: Human Resources. Retrieved from http://humanresources.about.com/cs/strategicplanning1/a/strategicplan.htm

Kelly-Thomas, K. J. (1998). *Clinical and nursing staff development: Current competence, future focus* (2nd ed.). Philadelphia: Lippincott.

Penn, B. K. (2008). *Mastering the teaching role: A guide for nurse educators.* Philadelphia: F.A. Davis.

3

Principles of Education

BACKGROUND

- *Teaching* is an art and science in which structured, sequenced information and experiences are transmitted to produce learning.
- *Learning* occurs when an individual changes behavior, mental processing, or emotional functioning as a result of exposure to new knowledge or experience (Braungart & Braungart, 2008).
- *Andragogy* is the art and science of teaching adults.
- Fundamental principles that guide the planning, implementation, and evaluation of adult education include:
  - Lifelong learning is the learner's responsibility.
  - Lifelong learning is essential to maintain competence.
  - Competence is critical to the delivery of quality, appropriate patient care.
  - The nursing professional development educator acts as a facilitator who actively partners with the learner during educational activities.
  - The nursing professional development educator is responsible for considering adult learning principles in planning and implementing educational activities that meet the needs of the organization and its employees.
  - Various formats are used to deliver educational activities to accommodate the diverse learning styles, learning needs, and characteristics of nurse populations.

- The nursing professional development educator is responsible for evaluating the impact of learning activities on the organization, job performance, and patient care (American Nurses Association, 2000).

PRINCIPLES OF ADULT EDUCATION

- Adults need a reason for learning.
  - Adults want to know from a personal perspective why it is important to attend an educational activity.
  - Communicating evidence that supports the need for an educational program is essential. Adults have the right and responsibility to know the rationale for attending educational activities.
- Adults are self-directed learners responsible for their own learning.
  - Self-direction in adults stems from a desire to have control over what they learn and how they learn it.
  - Adults participate in the planning, implementation, and evaluation of educational activities.
  - Adults participate in assessing educational needs.
- Adults bring varied life experiences to learning situations.
  - Life experiences may enhance learning even if they do not directly relate to the program topic.
  - Adult learners should be encouraged to share their life experiences if they are willing to do so.
  - The nursing professional development educator facilitates learning by helping learners apply their personal experiences to enhance the learning process.
- Adults are life-oriented learners. They focus on obtaining knowledge and skills that will help them in their daily lives.
  - Adults need to understand how specific knowledge, skills, and behaviors will benefit them in job performance, interpersonal interactions, and/or professional development.
  - Adults become impatient if they are forced to participate in educational activities that they believe are not purposeful or beneficial to work or their personal lives.
  - Adults approach education from a task-, problem-, or life-oriented perspective.
- Adults respond to both intrinsic and extrinsic motivators.
  - Motivators are factors perceived to be of benefit to the learner.
  - Examples of extrinsic motivators include salary increases, promotions, improved working conditions, and public recognition.
  - Examples of intrinsic motivators include increased self-esteem, ability to enhance interpersonal relationships, and enhanced job satisfaction.
  - Adults are more responsive to intrinsic motivators. Connecting educational program purpose to the adult learner's intrinsic motivators increases learning.
  - Nursing professional development educators must consider internal and external motivators when planning learning activities (Avillion, 2008).

LEARNING THEORIES

Behavioral Learning Theory

- Behavioral learning theory is based on the premise that all behavior is learned and can be influenced through the use of incentives or punishments to reach desired ends.
- This theory focuses on overt, measurable, observable behavior.
- Also called the S-R mode of learning, this theory suggests that learning occurs in response to altered stimulus conditions in the environment and/or reinforcement after a response.
- Behavioral theory applies the principles of respondent conditioning (responses are conditioned or unconditioned reflexes) and operant conditioning (desired behavior is reinforced to encourage the frequency of a desired response) to the learning situation.
- Transfer of learning occurs through repeated practice and consistent, immediate reinforcement.
- The educator's role is to arrange the environment, including the reinforcement, to produce desired behavior change and eliminate undesirable behavior (Vandeveer, 2009).

Cognitive Learning Theory

- Cognitive learning theory states that learning is a highly active process directed by the learner who uses cognitive skills to acquire and apply new information.
- This theory focuses on reorganizing information into new insights or understanding.
- According to this theory, goals and expectations within the individual create disequilibrium that produces the motivation for learning.
- The learner controls transfer of learning through information processing and application.
- Recognizing the learners' past experiences, perceptions, ways of processing information, and social influences that affect any learning situation is the focus of the educator.
- The educator's role is to consider available information about the learners when organizing and presenting the educational content (Braungart & Braungart, 2008; Vandeveer, 2009).

Social Learning Theory

- Social learning theory combines principles from behavioral and cognitive theories to propose that learning occurs in the context of social situations.
- This theory focuses on learning as a social process.
- Role modeling is a central concept of this theory: other people's behaviors provide compelling examples of how to think, feel, or act.
- This theory includes four phases: attention (observation of the role model), retention (processing in memory), reproduction (performance of observed actions), and motivation (reinforcement and/or punishment).
- Transfer of learning occurs as a result of repeated exposure to positive role models.
- The educator's role is to act as an exemplary role model and select socially healthy experiences for learners to observe (Braungart & Braungart, 2008).

Psychodynamic Learning Theory

- Psychodynamic learning theory emphasizes emotion and the importance of both conscious and unconscious forces in guiding behavior.
- This theory focuses on learning as an emotional process that is part of psychological growth and human development.
- Based on the work of Sigmund Freud, this theory often is considered a motivational theory that addresses emotion rather than cognition.
- Transfer of learning occurs through the learner's insights and the teacher–learner relationship.
- The educator's role is to work with learners to make unconscious motivations conscious and support the development of ego strength (Braungart & Braungart, 2008).

Humanistic Learning Theory

- Humanistic learning theory is based on the belief that each person is unique, autonomous, and wants to grow in a positive way.
- This theory focuses on the development of the individual, especially the emotional and affective personality components.
- According to this theory, self-direction and individual life experiences are essential to the process of learning.
- Self-evaluation, internal motivation, self-concept, and self-discovery are all important to the humanistic learning process.
- The ultimate goal of learning is to promote the development of self-actualization.
- The educator's role is to facilitate learning, not to serve as the source of all information (Braungart & Braungart, 2008; Vandeveer, 2009).

Multiple Intelligences Theory

- Multiple intelligences theory, based on the work of Howard Gardner, proposes that each individual possesses a unique profile of eight intelligences that forms the basis for learning throughout life.
- This theory focuses on biopsychosocial potentials that work together to promote individual learning and development, problem-solving, and interaction with the environment.
- The intelligences that work together to produce learning are bodily kinesthetic, visual–spatial, verbal-linguistic, logical-mathematical, musical-rhythmic, interpersonal, intrapersonal, and naturalist. Existential intelligence and moral intelligence are two other areas that Gardner suggested be studied further before adding them to the list of intelligences.
- Learners who identify their personal profile of intelligences can use that self-awareness to actively participate in creating a positive learning experience.
- The educator's role is to use knowledge of learners' profiles and/or the intelligences themselves to design meaningful learning experiences (Lowenstein & Bradshaw, 2001; Vandeveer, 2009).

CHARACTERISTICS OF ADULT LEARNERS

- Educators of adults have a responsibility to consider the characteristics of adult learners in planning, implementing, and evaluating learning experiences (Alspach, 1995; Bastable, 2008; Ellis & O'Connell, 2009; Kelly-Thomas, 1998).
- Because adults are heterogeneous learners, educators will:
  - Involve learners in determining their own learning needs and how to meet them.
  - Expect and encourage differences of opinion and meaning.
  - Respect the unique perspective and background of each learner.
- Because adults have multiple responsibilities, educators will:
  - Recognize that other responsibilities may interfere with readiness, participation, or learning achievement.
  - Provide flexibility in scheduling, teaching strategies, and options for learning to make education convenient for adults.
  - Provide opportunities for adults to participate actively in all phases of the educational experience.
- Because adults bring various life and work backgrounds to the current educational experience, educators will:
  - Assess past experiences and incorporate them into the educational activity.
  - Value the knowledge and skills that learners bring from their backgrounds to an educational environment.
  - Use teaching strategies that build on past experiences.
  - Emphasize the relationship between past experiences and present content to encourage transfer of learning.
- Because adults may be less flexible as learners, educators will:
  - Be open-minded and adaptable in designing educational activities.
  - Help learners integrate new concepts with previous beliefs and perspectives.
  - Give learners time to work through new information, consider how new concepts fit, and reach their own conclusions.
- Because adults may have negative past learning experiences, educators will:
  - Provide frequent positive reinforcement.
  - Create a learning climate that is conducive to a positive educational experience.
  - Show confidence in the learner's abilities to acquire the necessary knowledge and skills to change behavior.
  - Give learners positive or constructive feedback about performance.
- Because adults are voluntary learners, educators will:
  - Assess the motivational factors that influence learner participation in the educational activity.
  - Maintain realistic expectations of learners based on their motivation for attending the educational activity.
  - Identify and respond to behavioral cues that suggest that learner's needs are not being met.
- Adults are problem-centered learners who respond to educators who:
  - Identify and meet the learner's priority needs.
  - Focus the educational content on concrete essentials that learners can apply to their own situations.
  - Use a problem-centered approach that relates educational content to real-life situations.

- Educators who recognize that adults are knowledgeable learners will:
  - Approach learners as peers who are knowledgeable colleagues.
  - Display mutual respect and a sense of collegiality in interactions with learners.
  - Encourage learners to experiment and learn from their mistakes when possible, but be available to support learners when needed.
  - Provide helpful, useful, clear information using realistic scenarios to illustrate content.
- Because most adults are self-directed in their learning, educators will:
  - Provide opportunities for learners to use their own goals and expectations to evaluate the effectiveness of the educational activity.
  - Respond to evaluation feedback to provide additional educational support or make changes in future educational activities.
- Because adults of different ages need varying degrees of support in learning, educators will:
  - Create a learning environment (e.g., seating, ventilation, lighting, acoustics) that is comfortable and conducive to learning for individuals with varied physical, mental, emotional, and social capabilities.
  - Check in with learners often to adjust the pace of learning activities or provide support as needed.
  - Arrange coverage of content so that the most complex or challenging material is addressed when learners are at peak performance (Alspach, 1995; Fischer, 2009).

Learning Styles

- Learning style preferences refer to the ways in which learners prefer to approach learning as well as the conditions under which they learn most effectively and efficiently (Alspach, 1995; Kitchie, 2008).
- Learning style may be influenced over time by factors such as the environment, life experiences, job changes and demands, and personality traits.
- Learning is more likely to occur at educational activities that are designed to correspond with the learning styles of the audience (Kitchie, 2008).

Six Learning Style Principles
1. Both the educator's teaching style and the learner's learning style can be identified.
2. Educators must avoid relying on teaching methods and tools that fit their own preferred styles.
3. Educators are most helpful when they assist learners in identifing their own learning style preferences and pursue educational activities that match those preferences.
4. Learners should have the chance to learn using their preferred learning style.
5. Learners should be encouraged to take advantage of opportunities to expand their learning style preferences.
6. Educators can develop educational activities that support each learning style (Kitchie, 2008).

Learning Style Inventories
- A learning style inventory is used to measure learner preferences in the modes of learning and the corresponding learning style (Abbruzzese, 1996; Lowenstein & Bradshaw, 2001; Fischer, 2009; Kitchie, 2008).

Kolb's Experiential Learning Model

- Kolb's Experiential Learning Model is based on the premise that adults refine their approaches to learning over time as they perceive and process information. Influencing factors include past experiences, current environmental demands, and heredity. This model emphasizes the way meaning is attached to experience, not just the collection of experiences.
- Kolb's model describes four styles of learning that are reflective of two dimensions: perception and processing.
- Four modes of learning are identified as steps in the learning cycle: concrete experience (feeling), reflective observation (watching), abstract conceptualization (thinking), and active experimentation (doing).
- Based on the learner's strengths in perception and processing through the four modes of learning, Kolb described these four learning styles:
  1. Diverger: The learner emphasizes concrete experience and reflective observation (feeling/watching). These learners are sensitive and interested in people.
  2. Assimilator: The learner combines reflective observation and abstract conceptualization (watching/thinking). These learners focus on ideas and concepts.
  3. Converger: The learner integrates abstract conceptualization and active experimentation (thinking/doing). These learners excel at deductive reasoning to address specific problems or find the best solutions.
  4. Accommodator: The learner uses active experimentation and concrete experience (doing/feeling). These learners are oriented to facts and use intuitive, trial-and-error methods (Kolb, 1984).

Sensory Learning

- Sensory learning style theories reflect the belief that learners have preferences for the senses that they find most effective in processing information.
- **Visual learners** learn best through visual stimuli in an otherwise passive environment. These learners are attracted to images, handouts, colorful presentations, and dialogue with imagery.
- **Auditory learners** prefer to learn through the spoken word. These learners prefer audiotapes, lectures, or interactive dialogue and respond well to verbal directions.
- **Aural learners** like to learn through sound and music. These learners prefer information within a musical context or background.
- **Verbal learners** use a combination of the written and spoken word to learn most effectively. These learners like to learn through debates, concept papers, and simulation.
- **Kinesthetic learners** learn through hands-on involvement and physical activities. These learners learn most effectively through skill demonstrations, simulation, and experiential activities.
- The VARK (Visual-Auditory-Read/Write-Kinesthetic) is one tool that measures sensory learning styles (Avillion, 2008; Fischer, 2009; Kitchie, 2008).

Hemispheric Dominance

- *Hemispheric dominance, or right-brain/left-brain and whole-brain thinking,* emphasizes the specialized functions of the brain hemispheres as the source of learning preferences.
- The left hemisphere is the vocal and analytical side, used for speaking and logical thinking.

- The right hemisphere is the emotional, visual–spatial, and nonverbal side, used for artistic expression and creative thinking.
- Tools for measuring hemispheric dominance include the Brain Preference Indicator (BPI) and the Herrmann Brain Dominance Instrument (HBDI; Kitchie, 2008).

Benner's Novice to Expert Model

- Benner's Novice to Expert Model of Skill Acquisition describes how nurses acquire practice skills and knowledge.
- According to this model, skill acquisition is dependent on the learner's knowledge and experience over time.
- The five levels of nursing practice are:
  1. Novice (0 to 6 months): The learner has limited background and experience so rules govern behavior.
  2. Advanced beginner (6 months to 2 years): The learner has some experience but still needs extensive guidance.
  3. Competent (2 to 3 years): The learner has a sense of mastery and is able to perform adequately on a day-to-day basis unless major variations occur.
  4. Proficient (4 to 5 years): The learner perceives global aspects of situations, recognizes variations, and knows how to modify plans appropriately.
  5. Expert (5 to 7 years): The learner intuitively grasps each situation and problem-solves creatively and effectively (Benner, 1984; Fischer, 2009).

VARIATIONS IN LEARNER CHARACTERISTICS

Generational Differences

- Currently, the workforce is composed of four generations, each with its own set of characteristics, values, and preferences.
- Since educators often deal with audiences that include individuals from all four generations, a variety of activities can be used to address some of the needs and preferences of each generation.
- *Veterans* (born between 1926 and 1945) are products of the Great Depression and World War II. Veterans want recognition for their extensive knowledge and experience. They value tradition, hard work, and adherence to rules. As learners, veterans respect educators as authority figures and prefer formal learning environments and experiences (Avillion, 2009; Zager, 2008).
- *Baby Boomers* (born between 1946 and 1964) are the result of the postwar population growth and currently comprise almost half of the workforce. They enjoy learning, have a passion to achieve success, and want to make a difference in the world. Baby boomers value teamwork and personal gratification in the workplace. As learners, baby boomers respond best when treated as equals and exposed to open sharing of personal examples and interactive or team activities (Avillion, 2009; Zager, 2008).

- *Generation Xers* (born between 1965 and 1980) are often referred to as the "latch-key generation." Their values were shaped by events including political scandals like Watergate and societal trends like single-parent families. They value work-life balance, flexibility, and loyalty to self. As learners, Gen Xers prefer self-directed learning on their terms and stimulating visual or live activities that are fun (Avillion, 2008; Wellman, 2009; Zager, 2008).
- *Generation Yers* (born between 1981 and 2002) have grown up in a technological era, are globally oriented, and are comfortable with diversity. They are highly motivated and recognize that knowledge and skills increase their job marketability. This is important because they have little company loyalty. As learners, Gen Yers enjoy varied educational strategies and opportunities to interact with others for discussions or projects (Avillion, 2008; Wellman, 2009; Zager, 2008).

Cultural Diversity

- Because cultural diversity is a valued social and demographic part of society, nursing professional development educators work with learners who represent a variety of cultures.
- Culture is defined as the socially transmitted behavioral patterns, arts, beliefs, values, customs, and other characteristics of a group that guide their worldview and actions.
- Cultural competence is the process of integrating awareness of one's own knowledge, attitudes, beliefs, and skills with those from other cultures to enhance communication and interactions with others (Andrews, 2008b).
- Acculturation refers to the process of learning another culture and modifying one's own behavior following exposure to that culture.
- Assimilation is the process in which people from a nondominant culture adopt the behaviors and attitudes of the dominant culture (Husting, 2009).
- The cultural values and beliefs of learners influence the educational process and learning outcomes because they affect the learner's thinking, decisions, and actions (Husting, 2009).
- Cultural factors to consider in planning, implementing, and evaluating educational activities include verbal and nonverbal communication patterns and barriers; learning style preferences; beliefs and values; gender, interpersonal, and social roles; and time orientation (Andrews, 2008a).

REFERENCES

Abruzzese, R. S. (Ed.). (1996). *Nursing staff development: Strategies for success.* St. Louis, MO: Mosby.

Alspach, J. G. (1995). *The educational process in nursing staff development.* St. Louis, MO: Mosby.

American Nurses Association. (2000). *Scope and standards of practice for nursing professional development.* Silver Spring, MD: American Nurses Publishing.

Andrews, M. M. (2008a). Cultural diversity in the health care workforce. In M. M. Andrews & J. S. Boyle (Eds.), *Transcultural concepts in nursing care* (5th ed., pp. 297–326). Philadelphia: Lippincott Williams & Wilkins.

Andrews, M. M. (2008b). Culturally competent nursing care. In M. M. Andrews & J. S. Boyle (Eds.), *Transcultural concepts in nursing care* (5th ed., pp. 15–33). Philadelphia: Lippincott Williams & Wilkins.

Avillion, A. E. (2008). *A practical guide to staff development: Evidence-based tools and techniques for effective education* (2nd ed.). Marblehead, MA: HCPro.

Bastable, S.B. (2008). *Nurse as educator: Principles of teaching and learning for nursing practice.* Boston: Jones & Bartlett.

Benner, P. (1984). *From novice to expert: Excellence and power in clinical practice.* Menlo Park, CA: Addison-Wesley.

Braungart, M. M., & Braungart, R. G. (2008). Applying learning theories to healthcare practice. In S. B. Bastable (Ed.), *Nurse as educator: Principles of teaching and learning for nursing practice* (3rd ed., pp. 51–89). Boston: Jones & Bartlett.

Ellis, N. F., & O'Connell, K. M. (2009). Principles of adult learning. In S. L. Bruce (Ed.), *Core curriculum for staff development* (3rd ed., pp. 33–66). Pensacola, FL: National Nursing Staff Development Organization.

Fischer, K. J. (2009). Teaching learning methodologies. In S. L. Bruce (Ed.), *Core curriculum for staff development* (3rd ed., pp. 223–250). Pensacola, FL: National Nursing Staff Development Organization.

Husting, P. M. (2009). Cultural diversity and competence. In S. L. Bruce (Ed.), *Core curriculum for staff development* (3rd ed., pp. 181–193). Pensacola, FL: National Nursing Staff Development Organization.

Kelly-Thomas, K. J. (1998). *Clinical and nursing staff development: Current competence, future focus* (2nd ed.). Philadelphia: Lippincott.

Kitchie, S. (2008). Determinants of learning. In S. B. Bastable (Ed.), *Nurse as educator: Principles of teaching and learning for nursing practice.* (3rd ed., pp. 93–145). Boston: Jones & Bartlett.

Kolb, D. A. (1984). *Experiential learning: Experience as the source of learning and development.* Englewood Cliffs, NJ: Prentice-Hall.

Lowenstein, A. J., & Bradshaw, M. J. (2001). *Fuszard's innovative teaching strategies in nursing* (3rd ed.). Gaithersburg, MD: Aspen.

Vandeveer, M. (2009). From teaching to learning: Theoretical foundations. In D. M. Billings & J. A. Halstead. (Eds.), *Teaching in nursing: A guide for faculty* (3rd ed., pp. 189–226). St. Louis, MO: Saunders.

Wellman, D. S. (2009). The diverse learning needs of students. In D. M. Billings & J. A. Halstead (Eds.), *Teaching in nursing: A guide for faculty* (3rd ed., pp. 18–32). St. Louis, MO: Saunders.

Zager, L. R. (2008). Intergenerational perspectives. In B. K. Penn (Ed.), *Mastering the teaching role: A guide for nurse educators* (pp. 65-75). Philadelphia: F. A. Davis.

4

Domains of Learning

BACKGROUND

- Benjamin Bloom and other experts in educational psychology developed and published a taxonomy of educational objectives in 1956.
- Bloom's taxonomy is easy to understand and implement, and therefore, is widely used in the development, implementation, and evaluation of educational activities.
- The taxonomy provides a systematic, practical tool for educators to determine educational objectives based on levels of behavior in the learning process.
- The taxonomy is divided into three major classifications or domains of learning: cognitive, affective, and psychomotor (Bastable & Doody, 2008; Kelly-Thomas, 1998; Penn, 2008).
- Each classification is subdivided into specific hierarchical categories that reflect simple to complex desired outcomes.
- Achievement of complex outcomes is based on the successful integration of simple outcomes to form new behaviors.
- Although the domains of learning are classified as separate entities, they are actually interdependent domains that learners may experience simultaneously (e.g., thinking processes influence psychomotor performance; adopted values affect thinking processes; Scheckel, 2009).

- Educators must consider the interdependence of the domains of learning when planning educational objectives and activities.
- The implementation of a taxonomy based on domains of learning makes it possible for educators and learners to clearly and consistently delineate desired learning outcomes.
- Specific verbs, such as "demonstrate," appear in more than one domain of learning. When developing objective statements, both the verb and the content area for which performance is directed specify the learning domain and level.
- During the 1990s, a group of cognitive psychologists led by Lorin Anderson updated the taxonomy by renaming and reordering the categories in the cognitive domain (Armstrong, 2009; Clark, 2009; Overbaugh & Schultz, 2010).
- Some educators have revised the terminology of Bloom's taxonomy to knowledge (cognitive), skills (psychomotor), and attitude (affective), also referred to as KSA (McManus, 2009).

Relevance to Nursing Professional Development Practice

- According to the American Nurses Association (2000, p. 14), "learning activity content is individualized to the target audience, the resources available, and the domains of learning."
- The taxonomy serves as the foundation for writing measurable learning objectives that clearly identify the desired outcomes of the learning process.
- Appropriate learning objectives facilitate the selection of teaching strategies and identification of resources needed for successful completion of learning activities.
- Measurable learning objectives facilitate the evaluation process by clearly describing expected learning outcomes.

Cognitive Domain

- The cognitive domain (ways of knowing) refers to the development of intellectual skills or thinking processes.
- Learning in the cognitive domain involves the acquisition of facts and knowledge and making use of that knowledge.
- The cognitive domain includes six levels of behaviors. The levels, listed in order from simplest to most complex, are **knowledge, comprehension, application, analysis, synthesis,** and **evaluation.**
- Behaviors at each level must be mastered before progressing to the next higher level of behaviors (Hardigan, Cohen, & Hagen, 2006; Scheckel, 2009).
- **Knowledge** level objectives involve the recognition or recall of basic facts or information.
  - Verbs that measure **knowledge** are *define, describe, identify, list,* and *state.*
  - Example: After attending this program, the learner will describe the signs and symptoms of myasthenia gravis.
- Objectives that measure the **comprehension** level reflect the ability of the learner to interpret the meaning of knowledge and understand instructions or directions.
  - Verbs used to measure **comprehension** include *explain, distinguish, summarize, predict,* and *interpret.*
  - Example: After completing this learning module, the learner will explain the pathophysiology of respiratory acidosis, respiratory alkalosis, metabolic acidosis, and metabolic alkalosis.

- Objectives for the next level of behavior, **application**, refer to the use of an acquired concept in a specific situation.
  - Verbs that measure **application** include *differentiate, apply, use, prepare,* and *operate.*
  - Example: Following this learning lab session, the learner will use the standard algorithm for fluid replacement needs to calculate fluid administration amounts for a patient undergoing a surgical procedure.
- The fourth level of cognitive behavior, **analysis**, involves separation of concepts or information into parts and determining the relationships among the parts.
  - Verbs that may be used to measure **analysis** are *analyze, differentiate, relate, compare,* and *contrast.*
  - Example: At the conclusion of this learning activity, the learner will compare the effectiveness of different skin care products on wounds.
- The next level, **synthesis**, refers to the creation of new knowledge or meaning by combining diverse concepts and elements.
  - Objectives for this level may be measured with verbs such as *create, combine, design, generate,* and *revise.*
  - Example: After attending this educational seminar, the learner will create a clinical orientation plan for a novice RN.
- The highest level of cognitive behavior, **evaluation**, involves making value judgments about situations, ideas, or materials.
  - Verbs that may be used to measure the **evaluation** level include *judge, critique, defend, justify,* and *appraise.*
  - Example: After participation in this simulation exercise, the learner will critique the performance of team members in an emergency situation (Clark, 2009; Hardigan, Cohen, & Hagen, 2006; McManus, 2009).
- Methods commonly used to promote learning in the cognitive domain include lecture, individualized instruction (e.g., preceptorship, mentorship, skills training) and independent study activities (e.g., Web-based learning, journaling, learning modules; Bastable & Doody, 2008; McManus, 2009).

Affective Domain

- The affective domain (ways of feeling) refers to the way learners deal with emotional aspects or feelings.
- Learning in the affective domain involves internalization or commitment to feelings, values, beliefs, interests, and attitudes.
- The affective domain includes five categories of behaviors that specify the depth of the learner's emotional responses. The levels, listed in order from simplest to most complex, are **receiving phenomena, responding to phenomena, valuing, organizing,** and **internalizing values.**
- Behaviors at each level build on previous levels as the learner internalizes feelings, leading to personal growth and a shift from an external to an internal locus of control (Scheckel, 2009).
  - Objectives at the **receiving phenomena** level describe the learner's awareness or willingness to attend to data or receive a stimulus.
  - Verbs that measure **receiving phenomena** include *name, share, accept, select,* and *describe.*
  - Example: After attending a cultural diversity workshop, the learner will share personal perspectives about cultural influences in the workplace.

- The second level of the affective domain, **responding to phenomena**, is addressed by objectives that reflect active learner participation and involvement in a particular situation or phenomenon.
  - **Responding to phenomena** is measured using verbs such as *participate, perform, comply, present,* and *verbalize.*
  - Example: On completion of this learning module, the learner will participate in a debate about the significance of ethical principles in a clinical nursing situation.
- **Valuing**, the next level, is based on internal values and beliefs that are exhibited in behaviors and responses. Objectives for **valuing** reflect the behaviors and responses that demonstrate the worth or value a person attaches to an object, behavior, situation, or phenomenon.
  - Verbs that may be used to assess valuing include *demonstrate, volunteer, initiate, justify,* and *defend.*
  - Example: After attending this experiential learning workshop, the learner will demonstrate effective use of debriefing skills to promote learning through simulation.
- The next level of the affective domain, **organizing**, involves prioritizing values and placing them in a hierarchy of importance to create a unique value system.
  - Verbs that may be used to measure **organizing** are *compare, challenge, formulate, synthesize,* and *prioritize.*
  - Example: After participating in this seminar, the learner will challenge barriers to practice for advanced practice nurses.
- At the highest level of the affective domain, **internalizing values**, the learner integrates a value system that guides the learner's behavior.
  - The **internalizing values** level is measured using verbs such as *propose, validate, verify, act,* and *influence.*
  - Example: Upon successful completion of this course, the learner will act according to the ethical code for nurses in their daily practice (Bastable & Doody, 2008; Hardigan, Cohen, & Hagen, 2006; McManus, 2009).
- Effective teaching strategies to promote learning in the affective domain include group activities that encourage self-exploration (e.g., case studies, debate, simulation, role play; Bastable & Doody, 2008).

Psychomotor Domain

- The psychomotor domain (ways of doing) refers to physical movement, coordination, and motor skills.
- Learning in the psychomotor domain involves acquiring gross and fine motor abilities and neuromuscular coordination to perform increasingly complex actions.
- Development of psychomotor skills requires practice and is measured in terms of speed, precision, distance, procedures, or techniques.
- The psychomotor domain includes five categories of behaviors. The levels, listed in order from simplest to most complex, are **imitation, manipulation, precision, articulation,** and **naturalization.**
- At the most basic level, **imitation**, objectives refer to the ability to replicate actions with allowance for some weakness and inconsistency in completing the action. Time and speed required are based on learner abilities.
  - Verbs used to measure **imitation** include *follow, select, describe, identify,* and *display.*
  - Example: After reviewing this video, the learner will select the steps necessary to connect the portable oxygen for patient transport.

- Objectives at the second level of the psychomotor domain, **manipulation**, relate to the ability to follow directions to perform specific psychomotor skills after instruction and practice. Coordination, speed, and time required to complete the task may vary.
  - Manipulation may be assessed using verbs such as show, perform, explain, adhere, and provide.
  - Example: Following a practice session in the skills lab, the learner will perform the procedural steps in medication administration.
- Objectives at the next level, **precision**, reflect that actions are carried out in a logical sequence with well-coordinated movements and few noncritical errors. Although coordination is evident at this level, time and speed required for completion are still variable.
  - Verbs that can be used to measure **precision** include *demonstrate, assemble, organize, fix,* and *construct.*
  - Example: After completing the training module on wound care, the learner will demonstrate wound care techniques in the clinical setting according to hospital procedure.
- The fourth level of the psychomotor domain is **articulation.** Objectives at this level refer to coordinated actions that are completed in a logical sequence with minimal errors. Coordination, time, and speed required are all within reasonable expectations.
  - Verbs that measure **articulation** include *use, complete, operate, design,* and *originate.*
  - Example: After completing a course and clinical experience on physical assessment techniques, the learner will complete a respiratory assessment using auscultation, palpation, and percussion skills.
- At the highest level of the psychomotor domain, **naturalization**, objectives describe actions that are completed automatically, virtually error-free, with coordinated movements, and consistent performance.
  - Verbs used to measure **naturalization** include *demonstrate, discriminate, create, manipulate,* and *form.*
  - Example: After successfully completing the requirements for a clinical practicum, the learner will demonstrate proficiency in management of the discharge planning process (Huitt, 2003; McManus, 2009; Scheckel, 2009).
- Teaching methods that may be used effectively for psychomotor skills include return demonstration, supervised clinical practice, simulation, and other experiential learning activities.

REFERENCES

American Nurses Association. (2000). *Scope and standards of practice for nursing professional development.* Silver Spring, MD: American Nurses Publishing.

Armstrong, P. (2009). *Bloom's taxonomy.* Retrieved from http://www.vanderbilt.edu/cft/resources/teaching_resources/theory/blooms.htm

Bastable, S. B., & Doody, J. A. (2008). Behavioral objectives. In S. B. Bastable (Ed.), *Nurse as educator: Principles of teaching and learning for nursing practice* (3rd ed., pp. 383-427). Boston: Jones & Bartlett.

Clark, D. (2009). *Bloom's taxonomy of learning domains: The three types of learning.* Retrieved from http://www.nwlink.com/~donclark/hrd/bloom.html

Hardigan, P. C., Cohen, S. R., & Hagen, K. P. (2006). *Bloom's taxonomy.* Retrieved from www.nova.edu/hpdtesting/ctl/forms/bloomstaxonomy.pdf

Huitt, W. (2003). The psychomotor domain. *Educational Psychology Interactive.* Valdosta, GA: Valdosta State University. Retrieved from http://www.edpsycinteractive.org/topics/behsys/psymtr.html

Kelly-Thomas, K. J. (1998). *Clinical and nursing staff development: Current competence, future focus* (2nd ed.). Philadelphia: Lippincott.

McManus, N. S. (2009). Domains of learning. In S. L. Bruce (Ed.), *Core curriculum for staff development* (3rd ed., pp. 67–85). Pensacola, FL: National Nursing Staff Development Organization.

Overbaugh, R. C., & Schultz, L. (2010). *Bloom's taxonomy.* Retrieved from http://www.odu.edu/educ/roverbau/Bloom/blooms_taxonomy.htm

Penn, B. K. (2008). How adults learn. In B. K. Penn (Ed.), *Mastering the teaching role: A guide for nurse educators* (pp. 3–18). Philadelphia: F. A. Davis.

Scheckel, M. (2009). Selecting learning experiences to achieve curriculum outcomes. In D. M. Billings & J. A. Halstead (Eds.), *Teaching in nursing: A guide for faculty* (3rd ed., pp. 154–172). St. Louis, MO: Saunders.

5

Ethical and Legal Issues

BACKGROUND

- *Ethics* is an area of study that examines values, actions, and choices to determine right and wrong. *Laws* are rules of conduct that are enforced by authority. Ethics and law often overlap (American Nurses Association [ANA], 2001; Springhouse, 2009).
- A code of ethics makes explicit the values, behaviors, and beliefs that govern appropriate behavior for members of a profession.
- According to the American Nurses Association (ANA, 2000, p. 18), "the nursing professional development educator's decisions and actions are based on ethical principles."
- The practice of nursing professional development includes ethical responsibilities to self, colleagues, and learners (Condon, 2008).
- The nursing professional development educator provides educational activities on current and emerging ethical topics, including patients' rights, autonomy, end-of-life issues, and confidentiality.
- Resources with information about ethical principles and standards that are relevant to nursing professional development include:
  - ANA's *Scope and Standards of Practice for Nursing Professional Development* (2000) identifies 13 criteria that measure how decisions and actions are based on ethical principle.
  - ANA's *Code of Ethics for Nurses With Interpretive Statements* (2001) describes nine provisions of the ethical obligations and duties of every nursing professional.

- ANA's *Guide to the Code of Ethics for Nurses: Interpretation and Application* (2008) provides background information and case examples for each of the ANA code provisions.
    - In addition, accrediting organization standards (e.g., The Joint Commission) and specialty association standards (e.g., National Nursing Staff Development Organization) identify ethical standards for nursing practice (ANA, 2000; Burrell, 2009).
- Nursing professional development educators adhere to all regional, state, and national laws and regulations as well as business and management policies and procedures (American Nurses Credentialing Center [ANCC], 2009).
- Nursing professional development educators practice in a manner consistent with professional practice standards and relevant statutes and regulations (ANA, 2000).

Ethical Accountability

- Ethical principles include:
    - Autonomy: the right of a competent individual to self-govern or to exercise self-determination
    - Veracity: telling the truth
    - Confidentiality: protecting of personal information
    - Nonmaleficence: avoiding harm to and for one's client
    - Beneficence: doing good to and for one's client
    - Justice: fair distribution of resources to all members of society (Nelson, 2008)
- Ethical principles are woven throughout the ANA *Code of Ethics for Nurses* and other key documents that guide the practice of nursing professional development.
- The nine provisions of the ANA *Code of Ethics for Nurses* state that the nurse will:
    1. Practice with compassion and respect.
    2. Advocate for and be committed to the patient.
    3. Promote the health, safety, and rights of the patient.
    4. Maintain accountability for individual practice and appropriate delegation.
    5. Preserve integrity and safety.
    6. Improve healthcare environments and conditions of employment.
    7. Participate in advancement of the profession.
    8. Collaborate with others to meet health needs.
    9. Articulate nursing values and shape social policy (ANA, 2001).
- The nursing professional development educator is responsible for adhering to ethical principles in the assessment, planning, implementation, and evaluation of educational activities and in teacher–learner relationships (ANA, 2000).

Legal Accountability

- In the United States, each state has a nurse practice act, enacted by the state legislature, that defines the legal scope of nursing practice within that state. Each state also has a Board of Nursing that establishes and/or administers the rules and regulations for nursing practice (Springhouse, 2009).
- The nursing professional development educator practices within the legal scope of nursing as described by state nurse practice acts and state boards of nursing.

- The nursing professional development educator is legally responsible to maintain confidentiality within legal and regulatory parameters, safeguard learners' rights, and use appropriate standards and guidelines to guide practice (ANA, 2000).

Risk Management

- *Risk management* is a "process that identifies, analyzes, and treats potential hazards within a specific setting" (Guido, 2006).
- The purposes of risk management are to identify, analyze, treat, and evaluate actual or potential hazards that place an organization at risk and to eliminate or control potential risks to contribute to safe, quality-driven patient care (Dearmon, 2009).
- The risk management process relies on the analysis of data from patient events to determine root causes that can be addressed to prevent or minimize risk in the future.
- The nursing professional development educator is involved in risk management through role responsibilities and accountability for orientation, in-service training, continuing education, and competency assessment activities (Guido, 2006).

Boundary Issues

Conflict of Interest
- *Conflict of interest* exists when "an individual has an opportunity to affect continuing nursing education content in relation to a commercial interest with which he/she has a financial relationship" (ANCC, 2009).
- The nursing professional development educator has a responsibility to develop educational activities in a fair and unbiased manner.
- The educator must disclose the presence or absence of any potentially biasing relationship that may be perceived as a conflict of interest that might influence the content of an educational activity. A real or perceived conflict of interest must be identified early in the educational planning process and resolved prior to the implementation of the educational activity.

Intellectual Property
- *Intellectual property* refers to the ownership and proprietary rights that an individual or entity has for creations in the areas of copyrights, trademarks and servicemarks, patents, and trade secrets.
- The nursing professional development educator must deal appropriately with ethical dilemmas that arise related to intellectual property ownership. For example, if an educator creates a learning module in the course of employment, the intellectual property rights to the learning module belong to the employer. Therefore, the educator may not give or sell the learning module to any person or entity outside the organization (Burrell, 2009).

Plagiarism
- *Plagiarism* through inadequate citation of references or use of another's work without proper credit is a serious concern in educational activities.

- Strategies that may be used to avoid plagiarism include:
  - Use quotation marks to denote the exact wording of statements that come directly from a reference.
  - When paraphrasing from a reference, use your own words rather than rearranging or replacing a few words.
  - Be meticulous about citing references used in writing (Indiana University, 2004).
- If uncertain as to whether information should be cited, it is better to be cautious and cite it rather than risk accusations of plagiarism (Empire State College, 2010; Indiana University, 2004).

Cheating

- Other forms of educational dishonesty that the nursing professional development educator might encounter in practice include requests to falsify educational records (e.g., competency validation forms) or observation of cheating on a test. While these situations are difficult to address, the educator must adhere to both legal and ethical standards when they occur (ANA, 2000; Condon, 2008; Johnson, 2009; O'Shea & Robinson, 2002; Turner, 2002).

Confidentiality

- *Confidentiality* refers to the protection of information from or about an individual.
- The nursing professional development educator maintains confidentiality of learner and patient information throughout the educational process of assessment, planning, implementation, and evaluation (ANA, 2000).
- The educator may have access to personal information about learners as well as information from sources such as competency assessments, written exams, and progress evaluations. The educator should follow established policies and guidelines to protect the privacy and confidentiality of learner information (Johnson, 2009).

Copyright Law

- *Copyright* protects the original works of authorship in any tangible medium of expression, such as books, journal articles, sound or video recordings, music, art, plays, movies, computer software, and architecture (U.S. Copyright Office, 2009).
- Copyright does not protect:
  - Works that have not been fixed in a tangible form of expression, such as impromptu speeches or performances.
  - Titles, names, phrases, symbols, and slogans (although these may be protected as trademarks or servicemarks).
  - Ideas, procedures, processes, concepts, principles.
  - Works consisting of information that is common property, such as calendars, height and weight charts, and rulers (U.S. Copyright Office, 2008).
- Copyright occurs automatically when a work is created and fixed in a tangible form perceptible to others, such as a book, movie, or musical score.
- It is not necessary to register a work with the U.S. Copyright Office for the work to be protected, but registration is necessary to bring a lawsuit for infringement of an American work. Registration also is recommended to document copyright facts for public record and have a certificate as tangible record of registration.

- The copyright owner has exclusive rights to do and to authorize any of the following: reproduction or performance of copyrighted work, preparation of derivative works, or distribution of copies.
- The use of a copyright notice is not required for new works but may be beneficial since it informs the public that the work is protected by copyright, identifies the copyright owner, and shows the year of initial publication. The letter C within a circle, the word "Copyright," or the abbreviation "Copr" indicates copyright.
- It is not an infringement of copyright for a library, or any of its employees within the scope of their employment, to reproduce one copy of a work or to distribute a copy, if notice of copyright is included. If a hospital has a subscription to full text access, the subscription covers all employees. The fair use of a copyrighted work for purposes such as criticism, comment, news reporting, teaching (including multiple copies for classroom use), scholarship, or research, is not an infringement of copyright. In determining whether use in a specific situation constitutes fair use, four factors must be considered collectively:
  1. Purpose and character of the use, including whether such use is of a commercial nature or is for nonprofit educational purposes.
  2. Nature of the copyrighted material (e.g., fiction vs. nonfiction, published vs. unpublished).
  3. Amount and substantiality of the portion used in relation to the entire body of work (e.g., fair use for teaching is limited to copying of excerpts up to 1,000 words or 10% of a prose work, or the complete work, if less than 2,500 words; U.S. Copyright Office, 2009b).
  4. Effect of the use upon the potential market for or value of the work (U.S. Copyright Office, 2009a).
- Copyright issues of special interest to the nursing professional development educator relate to the use of materials in educational activities. Copyright law applies to the use of any original works of authorship including cartoons, charts, diagrams, graphics, photographs, and videos. Tangible use of any of these in presentations or handouts may violate copyright law unless written copyright permission is obtained. Citing the reference does not forego the need for permission (Burrell, 2009; O'Shea & Robinson, 2002; Turner, 2002; U.S. Copyright Office, 2009a).
- If uncertain as to whether use of intellectual property violates copyright, it is better to be cautious and obtain permission for use.

Regulatory Considerations

- The Americans With Disabilities Act (ADA) protects the rights of individuals with disabilities in the areas of employment and education (Frank, 2009).
- The ADA guarantees access to educational opportunities for individuals with physical and psychological disabilities, including learning disabilities (O'Shea & Robinson, 2002).
- The nursing professional development educator is responsible for making "reasonable accommodations" for learners to fully participate in educational activities (Gunby, 2008).

- The Occupational Safety and Health Administration (OSHA) is a division within the U.S. Department of Labor that exists to ensure safe and healthful conditions in the work environment by setting and enforcing standards and by providing training, outreach, education and assistance (OSHA, n.d.).
- OSHA regulations require healthcare employers to provide education on various topics related to health and safety, including H1N1, bloodborne pathogens, and universal precautions (Ellis & Hartley, 2008).
- The nursing professional development educator is involved in planning, implementing, and evaluating educational activities to meet OSHA mandates.
- The Pharmaceutical Research and Manufacturers of America (PhRMA) is an organization that represents pharmaceutical research and biotechnology companies. PhRMA works closely with the Food and Drug Administration (FDA) and supports the adverse drug event reporting process.
- In addition, PhRMA developed a *Code on Interactions with Healthcare Professionals* in collaboration with the Accreditation Council for Continuing Medical Education (ACCME). This code has become the basis for the standards for disclosure and commercial support in continuing nursing education activities (ANCC, 2009; PhRMA, 2009).
- The Family Educational Rights and Privacy Act (FERPA) is a federal law that addresses the privacy of student educational records (U.S. Department of Education, 2010).
- The nursing professional development educator must be familiar with FERPA regulations that allow students age 18 and older access to educational records. The law also requires written permission from the eligible student to release of information from a student's records except in specific, designated situations.
- The Clinical Laboratory Improvement Amendments (CLIA) program is administered by the Centers for Medicare & Medicaid Services to ensure quality laboratory testing on humans.
- The nursing professional development educator must be familiar with educational and competency requirements related to waived testing in clinical settings that were established by CLIA (Centers for Medicare & Medicaid Services, 2010).

Professional Standards

- *Professional standards* are statements, often developed by professional organizations, that reflect the values of a profession and describe behavioral expectations for individuals who practice in that profession (Ellis & Hartley, 2008).
- The ANA *Scope and Standards of Practice for Nursing Professional Development* describes the philosophy, framework, and roles of nursing professional development educators. *Scope and Standards* also delineates six standards of practice and nine standards of professional performance that define expected behaviors for an educator (ANA, 2000).
- ANCC, a separately incorporated subsidiary of ANA, provides credentialing programs for individuals and organizations in nursing. ANCC offers a certification program to recognize individual nurses in specialty practice areas, an accreditation program to accredit providers and approvers of continuing nursing education, and recognition programs to recognize healthcare organizations for promoting safe, positive work environments (ANCC, 2010).
- *Certification* is a voluntary "process by which a professional organization validates, based on predetermined standards, an individual registered nurse's qualifications, knowledge, and practice in a defined functional or clinical area of nursing" (ANA, 2000, p. 23).

- *Accreditation* is "a voluntary process in which an institution, organization, or agency submits to an in-depth analysis to determine its capacity to provide or approve quality continuing education over an extended period of time" (ANCC, 2009, p. 73).
- ANCC Commission on Accreditation is responsible for developing and administering the criteria and procedures that govern the process for accreditation of continuing nursing education.
- *Continuing education* is defined as a set of learning experiences designed to supplement the knowledge, skills, and attitudes of nurses, thereby enhancing quality health care and the pursuit of professional career goals (ANA, 2000).
- ANCC *accredited providers* are organizations or work units within organizations that plan, implement, and evaluate continuing nursing education activities that meet an established set of criteria.
- ANCC *accredited approvers* are organizations that meet an established set of approval criteria and approve educational activities, providers, or both. Accredited approvers fall into one of four categories: constituent member associations of ANA, specialty nursing organizations, federal nursing services, or national nursing organizations based outside the United States.
- The term *approved provider* is used to designate an organization or work unit within an organization that has been approved by an accredited approver to provide continuing nursing education activities.
- An approved provider and an accredited provider *cannot* approve continuing nursing education activities provided by another organization or institution (ANCC, 2009).

REFERENCES

American Nurses Association. (2000). *Scope and standards of practice for nursing professional development.* Washington, DC: American Nurses Publishing.

American Nurses Association. (2001). *Code of ethics for nurses with interpretive statements.* Washington, DC: American Nurses Publishing.

American Nurses Association. (2008). *Guide to the code of ethics for nurses: Interpretation and application.* Silver Spring, MD: Nursebooks.org.

American Nurses Credentialing Center. (2009). *Application manual: Accreditation program.* Silver Spring, MD: American Nurses Credentialing Center.

American Nurses Credentialing Center. (2010). *About ANCC.* Retrieved from http://www.nursecredentialing.org/FunctionalCategory/AboutANCC.aspx

Burrell, T. S. (2009). Ethical and legal principles. In S. L. Bruce (Ed.), *Core curriculum for staff development* (3rd ed., pp. 87–110). Pensacola, FL: National Nursing Staff Development Organization.

Centers for Medicare & Medicaid Services. (2010). *Clinical laboratory improvement amendments overview.* Retrieved from http://www.cms.gov/clia

Condon, E. H. (2008). Ethical issues in teaching nursing. In B. K. Penn (Ed.), *Mastering the teaching role: A guide for nurse educators* (pp. 401–410). Philadelphia: F. A. Davis.

Dearmon, V. (2009). Risk management and legal issues. In L. Rousell & R. C. Swansburg (Eds.), *Management and leadership for nurse administrators* (5th ed., pp. 470–493). Sudbury, MA: Jones & Bartlett.

Ellis, J. R., & Hartley, C. L. (2008). *Nursing in today's world* (9th ed.). Philadelphia: Lippincott, Williams & Wilkins.

Empire State College. (2010). *What is plagiarism and how to avoid it?* Retrieved from http://esclibrary.blogspot.com/2010/04/what-is-plagiarism-and-how-to-avoid-it.html

Frank, B. (2009). Teaching students with disabilities. In D. M. Billings & J. A. Halstead (Eds.), *Teaching in nursing: A guide for faculty* (3rd ed., pp. 53–72). St. Louis, MO: Saunders.

Guido, G. W. (2006). *Legal and ethical issues in nursing* (4th ed.). Upper Saddle River, NJ: Pearson Prentice Hall.

Gunby, S. S. (2008). Legal issues in teaching nursing. In B. K. Penn (Ed.), *Mastering the teaching role: A guide for nurse educators* (pp. 411–420). Philadelphia: F. A. Davis.

Indiana University (2004). *Plagiarism: What it is and how to recognize and avoid it.* Retrieved from http://www.indiana.edu/~wts/pamphlets/plagiarism.shtml

Johnson, E. G. (2009). The academic performance of students. In D. M. Billings & J. A. Halstead (Eds.), *Teaching in nursing: A guide for faculty* (3rd ed., pp. 33–52). St. Louis, MO: Saunders.

Nelson, M. J. (2008). Ethical, legal, and economic foundations of the educational process. In S. B. Bastable (Ed.), *Nurse as educator: Principles of teaching and learning for nursing practice* (3rd ed., pp. 25–49). Boston: Jones & Bartlett.

Occupational Safety and Health Agency. (n.d.). *About OSHA.* Retrieved from http://osha.gov/about.html

O'Shea, K. L., & Robinson, C. B. (2002). Legal and ethical issues in education. In K. L. O'Shea (Ed.), *Staff development nursing secrets* (pp. 59–63). Philadelphia: Hanley & Belfus.

Pharmaceutical Research and Manufacturers of America. (2009). *PhRMA statement before U.S. Senate special committee on aging.* Retrieved from http://www.phrma.org/phrma-statement-before-us-senate-special-committee-aging

Springhouse. (2009). *Evidence-based nursing guide to legal & professional issues.* Philadelphia: Lippincott Williams & Wilkins.

Turner, M. (2002). Legal and ethical concerns. In B. E. Puetz & J. W. Aucoin (Eds.), *Conversations in nursing professional development* (pp. 343–347). Pensacola, FL: Pohl Publishing.

U.S. Copyright Office. (2008). *Copyright basics.* Retrieved from http://www.copyright.gov/circs/circ1.pdf

U.S. Copyright Office. (2009a). *Copyright law of the United States and Related Laws Contained in Title 17 of the United States Code.* Retrieved from http://www.copyright.gov/title17/circ92.pdf

U.S. Copyright Office. (2009b). *Reproduction of copyrighted works by educators and librarians.* Retrieved from http://www.copyright.gov/circs/circ21.pdf

U.S. Department of Education. (2010). *Family educational rights and privacy act (FERPA).* Retrieved from http://www2.ed.gov/policy/gen/guid/fpco/ferpa/index.html

6

Issues and Trends

CONTINUED COMPETENCE

- According to the American Nurses Association (ANA, 2000, p. 23), *continuing competence* is the "ongoing professional nursing competence according to level of expertise, responsibility, and domains of practice as evidenced by behavior based on beliefs, attitudes, and knowledge matched to and in the context of a set of expected outcomes as defined by nursing scope of practice, policy, code of ethics, standards, guidelines, and benchmarks that ensure safe performance of professional activities."
- Competence begins with academic preparation, licensure, and initial competencies to perform one's job function. Ongoing competence reflects the new, changing, high-risk, and problematic aspects of the job role (Wright, 2005).

Academic Qualifications

- Professional development educators should have a graduate degree in nursing or a related specialty.
- If the graduate degree is in a related discipline (e.g., adult education), the baccalaureate degree must be in nursing.

- The graduate degree itself is determined by the role of the nursing professional development educator.
- If the educator's primary role is specialty or unit-based and she or he functions as both a patient care provider and an educator (e.g., clinical nurse specialist), it may be most appropriate to obtain a graduate degree in nursing with specialty emphasis.
- If the role is primarily that of educator with a focus on program development and implementation, it may be most appropriate to obtain a graduate degree in adult education.
- Professional development educators must demonstrate knowledge of essential education content; the most effective teaching and learning delivery methods; and the skills to plan, develop, implement, and evaluate learning activities.
- Persons who function as administrators of professional development departments should optimally possess a doctoral degree in nursing or a related field (e.g., adult education).
- One of the degrees of a nursing professional development administrator is to be in nursing (i.e., baccalaureate, master's degree, doctorate).
- Administrators must demonstrate not only knowledge of the education process but possess skills in management and business administration (ANA, 2000; Avillion, 2005).

Licensure

- Licensure is a mandatory process by a governmental agency to permit an individual to engage in a profession or occupation.
- Nursing practice is legally regulated by the definition of nursing in state nurse practice acts.
- Legal boundaries are based on interpretation of the safe practice of nursing according to these acts.
- State boards of nursing use nursing practice guidelines to issue licensure and protect the welfare of the public.
- Professional development educators are nurses who must be licensed and must practice according to the mandates and guidelines of their nurse practice acts (ANA, 2000).
- The nursing professional development educator is to be familiar with the state practice acts and other rules and regulations that apply to the roles he or she teaches.

Role Certification

- The ANA (2000, p. 34) *Scope and Standards of Practice* states, "the registered nurse in a nursing role specialty obtains and maintains professional certification if available in the area of expertise."
- Certification recognizes the nurse as having successfully completed an examination in a particular specialty, thereby acknowledging the possession of advanced knowledge.
- The American Nurses Credentialing Center (ANCC) offers a certification examination in nursing professional development.
- Examination candidates must hold a current, active, unrestricted professional RN license in the United States or its territories; hold a baccalaureate degree or higher in nursing; have a minimum of 4,000 hours of clinical practice in the specialty area within the past 5 years; and have completed 30 hours of continuing education in nursing professional development within the past 3 years.
- Certification is good for a term of 5 years, after which various recertification options are available (ANA, 2004; ANCC, 2010; Swails, 2009).

Scope and Standards of Practice for Nursing Professional Development

- The *Scope and Standards* establish the foundational competencies for the nursing professional development educator.
- The ANA first published standards pertaining to this specialty in 1974 as *Standards for Continuing Education in Nursing*; revisions were published as *Standards for Nursing Staff Development* in 1990 and *Standards for Nursing Professional Development: Continuing Education and Staff Development* in 1994.
- The *Scope and Standards* support the maintenance of high standards in the delivery of educational programs by "ensuring that qualified individuals provide nursing professional development and educational services" (ANA, 2000, p. vii).

Note. This publication is for the nursing professional development test content outline effective November 1, 2008, that incorporates the 2000 *Scope & Standards*. Newly adopted standards are spelled out in *Nursing Professional Development: Scope & Standards of Practice* (2010), which is expected to be incorporated in the next test content outline.

Mandatory Education

- Professional nurses are expected to be lifelong learners (ANA, 2000, 2004).
- To achieve and maintain competence, it is essential that all nurses participate in continuing education activities.
- Many states mandate a specific number of hours of continuing education to maintain licensure.
- Nurses who hold specialty certifications must participate in a specific number of hours of continuing education and/or meet other professional development requirements to obtain recertification (ANA, 2000; ANCC, 2010).

Portfolio Components

- A portfolio is "material documenting the professional development, career planning, demonstration of learning, and maintenance of continuing professional nursing competence of the individual nurse" (ANA, 2000, p. 25).
- Portfolios can be used for performance evaluation, promotion eligibility, pay increases or bonuses, and/or placement on a career ladder.
- The format of a portfolio can vary depending on institution or individual requirements. Components may include:
  - Curriculum vitae or resume
  - Academic preparation; unofficial transcripts, current coursework; copies of degree diploma(s)
  - Nonacademic education: conferences, specialized training, continuing education
  - Certification documents
  - Professional nursing organization(s) membership and activities
  - Volunteer activities for organization and community
  - Participation in shared governance, institution or department committees
  - Research and evidence-based practice

- Publications
- Teaching activities
- Special projects
- Awards, recognitions, supervisor recommendations (ANA, 2000; Brunt, 2002; Holecek & Foard, 2009)

PRACTICE AND EXCELLENCE INITIATIVES

- The nursing professional development educator provides educational activities that support an organization's adoption of policies and procedures related to healthcare industry initiatives.
- Committee and task force involvement provides the opportunity for the educator to participate in the design and roll-out of practice and excellence initiatives.
- Partnering with other experts in the organization eliminates departmental barriers and enhances the quality and usefulness of educational programs (Kelly-Thomas, 1998).

Institute for Healthcare Improvement (IHI)

- IHI is an independent, nonprofit organization aimed at leading the improvement of health care throughout the world.
- IHI has a number of programs for organizations to participate in or use to improve healthcare according to the Institute of Medicine's six improvement aims: safety, effectiveness, patient-centeredness, timeliness, efficiency, and equity.
- Examples of past and present programs include The 5 Million Lives Campaign; Improving Outcomes for High-Risk and Critically Ill Patients, which led to the ventilator and central line bundles, rapid response teams, and glucose control interventions; IHI Perinatal Bundles; and prevention of catheter-associated urinary tract infections (Institute for Healthcare Improvement, n.d.).

Transforming Care at the Bedside (TCAB)

- TCAB began as an initiative between IHI and the Robert Wood Johnson Foundation from 2003 to 2008. This initiative created a framework for change on medical/surgical units prompted by the Institute of Medicine's report, *To Err is Human*.
- Examples of TCAB change innovations include rapid-response teams, specific communication models among caregivers, redesigned work spaces, liberal diet plans and meal delivery for patients, and professional support programs such as preceptorships and educational opportunities.
- TCAB has become an IHI Collaborative. It is a nontraditional quality improvement program in that it is engaging frontline staff and unit managers to develop innovations and exemplary care models to improve outcomes for patients and staff.
- The framework for change has four main categories:
  - Safe and reliable care
  - Vitality and teamwork
  - Patient-centered care
  - Value-added care processes (Institute for Healthcare Improvement, n.d.)

Centers for Medicare & Medicaid Services (CMS)

- A major reimbursement source for hospitals, CMS began decreased reimbursement for nonadherence to quality performance measures in 2001.
- In 2008, CMS eliminated payment for 10 preventable hospital-acquired conditions:
  - Stage III and IV pressure ulcers
  - Fall or trauma resulting in serious injury
  - Vascular catheter–associated infection
  - Catheter-associated urinary tract infection
  - Foreign object retained after surgery
  - Certain surgical site infections
  - Air embolism
  - Blood incompatibility
  - Certain manifestations of poor blood sugar control
  - Certain deep vein thromboses or pulmonary embolisms
- CMS also has "never events," events that should never occur when a patient is being cared for in a hospital. Examples are wrong surgical site on patient, wrong surgery on patient, infant discharged with wrong person, retention of a foreign object in a patient after surgery or procedure, patient death resulting from a fall while being cared for in a hospital, and death or serious disability related to a medication error.
- Nursing care influences preventable hospital-acquired conditions and "never events." The NPD educator has a role in training staff on facility policies and nursing procedures to prevent them (Hines & Yu, 2009).

The Joint Commission National Patient Safety Goals

- "Founded in 1951, The Joint Commission seeks to continuously improve health care for the public, in collaboration with other stakeholders, by evaluating health care organizations and inspiring them to excel in providing safe and effective care of the highest quality and value" (The Joint Commission, 2009).
- National Patient Safety Goals (NPSG) were established in 2002 to assist hospitals to address specific patient safety concerns. The Joint Commission continues to focus NPSGs on high-priority topics in patient safety and quality care.
- A NPSG may be "retired" so the focus stays on the most critical issues. However, retired NPSGs often become part of the standards by which a facility is evaluated on for accreditation.
- 2010 NPSGs topics for hospitals are patient identification, improved communication, medication safety, reduction of health care–related infections, falls reduction, prevention of pressure ulcers, and identification of safety risks in patient populations (The Joint Commission, 2010).

The ANCC Magnet Recognition Program®

- The Magnet Program recognizes healthcare organizations for promoting safe, positive work environments that promote the profession of nursing and quality patient outcomes.
- Initial research in 1983 led to the identification of 14 Forces of Magnetism. A statistical review of data from 2005 led to a revised model that was introduced in 2008. The new model groups the 14 Forces of Magnetism into 5 Model Components:
    1. Transformational Leadership
    2. Structural Empowerment
    3. Exemplary Professional Practice
    4. New Knowledge, Innovation, & Improvements
    5. Empirical Quality Results
- Magnet is seen as a benchmark of quality care (ANCC, 2008a).

The ANCC Pathway to Excellence® Program

- The Pathway to Excellence program is a nursing practice excellence recognition that originated from the Texas Nurses Association's Texas Nurse-Friendly Program.
- Organizations show how guidelines, known as The Pathway to Excellence Standards, are integrated in operating policies, procedures, and management practices of the healthcare organization.
- Standards include:
    - Control of nursing practice
    - Safety of the work environment
    - Systems exist to address patient care concerns
    - Nurse orientation
    - Chief nursing officer
    - Professional development
    - Competitive wages
    - Nurse recognition
    - Balanced lifestyle
    - Exemplary interdisciplinary collaboration
    - Leadership accountability
    - Quality initiatives (Swartwout, 2009; Wood, 2009)

The ANCC Nursing Skills Competency Program

- "ANCC's Nursing Skills Competency Program addresses concerns regarding competency of the nurse by validating that a skills program meets national design standards" (ANCC, 2008b, p. 4).
- The Program can be used by hospitals, manufacturers or distributors of commercial healthcare products, universities and schools of nursing, temporary staffing agencies, and state nurses associations.
- The accreditation is for an educational program, not an organization.

- In addition to following the ANCC educational design criteria in continuing education, validity and reliability requirements and selection criteria for faculty also must be demonstrated.
- The Nursing Skills Competency Program is a national performance benchmark so nurses may transfer their competency validation from employer to employer (ANCC, 2008b).

CREDENTIALING

- Credentialing, according to The Joint Commission (2007, pp. 93–94) is "the process of obtaining, verifying, and assessing the qualifications of a health care practitioner to provide patient care services in or for a health care organization."
- An organization specifies the minimum credentials required for each job role within the organization.
- Credentials include evidence of education, licensure, training, experience, and certifications (The Joint Commission, 2007).

Certification

- Certification is a process by which a nongovernmental agency or an association validates an individual's knowledge, skills, and abilities in a defined role and clinical area of practice, based on predetermined standards.
- Certification can be voluntary or mandatory.
- "Certification can be used for entry into practice, validation of competence, recognition of excellence, and/or for regulation" (ANCC, 2010, p. 6).
- The certifying organization determines the educational credential for professional certification. For example, a baccalaureate in nursing is required for eligibility to take the certification examination in nursing professional development.
- The certifying organization also determines the credential that is used upon attaining certification, for example, RN-BC, CCRN.
- The Accreditation Board for Specialty Nursing Certification accredits nursing and associated certification programs. The National Commission for Certifying Agencies accredits certification programs and organizations that assess professional competence in the areas of public health, welfare, and safety.
- Examples of organizations that provide certification for nursing specialties are American Association of Critical-Care Nurses' Certification Corporation, American Nurses Credentialing Center, National Certification Corporation, and Oncology Nurses Credentialing Certification Corporation.
- The renewal process for certification, determined by the certification organization, typically requires continuing education (ANCC, 2010; Kelly-Thomas, 1998).

Certificates

- Certificates are obtained for clinical practice skills based on safety and standards of care. Examples include basic cardiac life support, neonatal resuscitation program, fetal heart-rate monitoring, and chemotherapy administration.
- These certificates require a renewal process demonstrating the skill to ensure competency is maintained.
- Nursing professional development educators often have the credentials to be instructors in programs that provide these certifications.
- Healthcare institutions may also establish standards by which staff are certified to perform specific skills within that organization such as IV insertion, Foley insertion, telemetry monitoring.
- The nursing professional development professional provides the training and validation of institution-based certification.

PRACTICE BASED ON EVIDENCE

Background

- Evidence-based practice (EBP) is a problem-solving method that integrates
  - the search and critical appraisal of relevant data to answer a clinical question,
  - one's own clinical expertise, and
  - the patient's preferences and values (Melnyk & Fineout-Overholt, 2005).
- Research utilization differs from EBP in that it uses knowledge typically based on a single study.
- EBP can be applied to the practice of nursing professional development by using data related to the practice of teaching, the educator's expertise, and learner characteristics.
- Content for educational programs is to be evidenced-based.

Five Steps of Evidence-Based Practice

- *Step 1:* Formulate the burning clinical question in the PICO format: Patient population, Intervention of interest, Comparison intervention or status, and Outcome.
- *Step 2:* Search for best evidence from a hierarchy of evidence.
- *Step 3:* Conduct a critical review of the evidence.
- *Step 4:* Integrate the evidence with the provider's expertise, assessment of the patient, available resources, and the patient's preferences.
- *Step 5:* Evaluate the effectiveness of the evidenced-based intervention in meeting the desired outcome (Melnyk & Fineout-Overholt, 2005).

Sources of Evidence

- **Literature:** Literature is one of the most accessible forms of evidence. Published literature can be limited due to researchers' failure to publish, a reluctance to share proprietary information, and English language journals typically preferring to publish positive findings (Malloch & Porter-O'Grady, 2006).
- **Databases:** Many databases with healthcare information can be accessed free of charge or for a fee from a vendor. Vendor access subscription is typically done via an organization. While there may be some overlap, each database has a specific focus. The most commonly used databases for clinical content are:
  - Cochrane Database of Systematic Reviews: Full text of regularly updated systematic reviews; contains seven different databases (http://www.cochrane.org).
  - National Guidelines Clearinghouse: Summaries of guidelines based on scientific evidence or consensus of expert opinion; supported by the Agency for Healthcare Research and Quality (AHRQ;http://www.guideline.gov).
  - PubMed: A catalog of more than 4,600 biomedical journals' citations, usually with abstracts (full text articles are available from journal vendors); produced by the National Library of Medicine; organized by medical subject headings as well as searchable by citation (http://www.ncbi.nlm.nih.gov/sites/entrez).
  - Cumulative Index of Nursing and Allied Health Literature (CINAHL): Citations with available abstracts from 13 nursing, allied health, and bioscience; includes journals, books, drug monographs, dissertations, and images (http://www.ebscohost.com/cinahl/).
  - PsycINFO: Scholarly literature including books and dissertations in behavioral sciences; available through American Psychological Association (APA) or Ovid (http://www.apa.org/pubs/databases/psycinfo/index.aspx; Melnyk & Fineout-Overholt, 2005).
  - Educational Resources Information Center (ERIC): Bibliographic records of journal articles and other education-related materials (http://www.eric.ed.gov/).
  - Quality and Safety Education for Nurses (QSEN): Funded by the Robert Wood Johnson Foundation, QSEN has annotated bibliographies and teaching strategies essential to the development of quality and safety competencies (http://www.qsen.org/).
- **Reliable sources:** Clinical trials are one of the most reliable sources, although results need to be generalizable to the current situation. Source credibility can be based on past accomplishments, publications in peer-reviewed journals, and association with specialty organizations (Malloch & Porter-O'Grady, 2006; Melnyk & Fineout-Overholt, 2005).
- **Expert opinion:** Expert opinion can be used as an adjunct to research data, or when there is a lack of or conflict in research-based studies. Expert opinion can be found at conferences, professional Web sites, or from clinical experts (Malloch & Porter-O'Grady, 2006).
- **Best practices:** Best practices are protocols and practices based on standards that have quality clinical and financial outcomes (Malloch & Porter-O'Grady, 2006)

REFERENCES

American Nurses Association. (2000). *Scope and standards of practice for nursing professional development*. Washington, DC: American Nurses Publishing.

American Nurses Association. (2004). *Nursing scope and standards of practice*. Washington, DC: American Nurses Publishing.

American Nurses Credentialing Center. (2008a). *A new model for ANCC's Magnet Recognition Program* [Brochure]. Silver Spring, MD: Author.

American Nurses Credentialing Center. (2008b). *Overview of ANCC Nursing Skills Competency Program: A new kind of nursing accreditation* [Brochure]. Silver Spring, MD: Author.

American Nurses Credentialing Center. (2010). *2010 general testing and renewal handbook*. Silver Spring, MD: Author.

Avillion, A. E. (2005). *Nurse educator manual: Essential skills and guidelines for effective practice*. Marblehead, MA: HCPro.

Brunt, B. A. (2002). Standards of practice. In B. E. Puetz & J. W. Aucoin (Eds.), *Conversations in nursing professional development* (pp. 365–372). Pensacola, FL: Pohl Publishing.

Hines, P. A., & Yu, K. M. (2009). The changing reimbursement landscape: Nurses' role in quality and operational excellence. *Nursing Economic$, 27*(1), 7–13.

Holecek, A., & Foard, M. (2009). Promoting a culture of professionalism: The birth of the nursing portfolio. *Nurse Leader, 7*(6), 30–35.

Institute for Healthcare Improvement. (n.d.). *IHI.org: A resource from the Institute for Healthcare Improvement*. Retrieved from http://www.ihi.org/ihi/programs

Joint Commission, The. (2009). *Facts about The Joint Commission* [Fact Sheet]. Retrieved October 2, 2010, from http://www.jointcommission.org/AboutUs/Fact_Sheets/joint_commission_facts.htm

Joint Commission, The. (2010). *2010 National patient safety goals* [PowerPoint slides]. Retrieved from http://www.jointcommission.org/NR/rdonlyres/868C9E07-037F-433D-8858-0D5FAA4322F2/0/July2010NPSGs_Scoring_HAP2.pdf

Joint Commission Resources. (2007). *Assessing hospital staff competencies* (2nd ed.). Oakbrook Terrace, IL: Joint Commission on Accreditation of Healthcare Organizations.

Kelly-Thomas, K. J. (1998). *Clinical and nursing staff development: Current competence, future focus* (2nd ed.). Philadelphia : Lippincott.

Malloch, K., & Porter-O'Grady, T. (2006). *Introduction to evidence-based practice in nursing and health care*. Boston : Jones & Bartlett.

Melnyk, B. M., & Fineout-Overholt, E. (2005). *Evidence-based practice in nursing & healthcare: A guide to best practice*. Philadelphia : Lippincott Williams & Wilkins.

Swails, S. (2009). Issues and trends. In S. L. Bruce (Ed.), *Core curriculum for staff development* (3rd ed., pp. 139-159). Pensacola, FL: National Nursing Staff Development Organization.

Swartwout, E. (2009). *ANCC's Pathway to Excellence program*. Silver Spring, MD: American Nurses Credentialing Center. Retrieved from http://www.nursecredentialing.org/Pathway/ProgramOverview/Background-and-Overview.aspx

Wood, D. (2009). *ANCC's Pathway to Excellence: Commitment to good nursing environments*. AMN Healthcare. Retrieved from http://www.nursezone.com/Nursing-News-Events/more-features/ANCC%E2%80%99s-Pathway-to-Excellence-Commitment-to-Good-Nursing-Environments_32216.aspx

Wright, D. (2005). *The ultimate guide to competency assessment in health care* (3rd ed.). Minneapolis, MN: Creative Health Care Management, Inc.

7

Functions of the Nursing Professional Development Specialty

BACKGROUND

- "Educators develop, plan, and present educational activities…(that) directly or indirectly foster the development of competence in the learner" (American Nurses Association [ANA], 2000, p. 8).
- In the educator role, nursing professional development educators provide orientation, inservice, and continuing education.
- Orientation includes preceptor development and competency assessment, in addition to learning activities to help new employees learn their roles within the organization.
- Inservice entails using different teaching methods to educate staff on how to perform in their roles within the organization.
- Continuing education involves educational activities that are designed to enhance knowledge, skills, or attitudes regardless of the participant's employer.

ORIENTATION

- Orientation is "the process of introducing nursing staff to the philosophy, goals, policies, procedures, role expectations, and other factors needed to function in a specific work setting" (ANA, 2000, p. 25).
- Orientation occurs for employees new to an organization and when an employee changes roles, responsibilities, and/or practice settings within an organization.
- Aspects of orientation include job description; organizational and departmental policies and procedures; information management; performance improvement process; regulatory requirements; patient population-specific considerations; and competency assessment for role-specific duties, documentation, and equipment (Kelly-Thomas, 1998; O'Shea, 2002).
- The length of orientation varies according to the knowledge, skills, and abilities required for the position and the experience of the employee.
- Role transition requires that the employee learns the values, expected behaviors, and essential knowledge to perform her or his role competently in the organization (O'Shea, 2002).
- "New nursing staff members' competence is assessed, validated, and developed in orientation" (ANA, 2000, p. 5).
- Developing competence is accomplished through "processes and programs designed to cultivate, generate, and extend the competence of nurses related to expectations and performance standards new to the person or new to the organization" (Kelly-Thomas, 1998, p. 26).
- "Competency-based education (CBE) is an alternative approach to instruction that emphasizes a learner's ability to demonstrate integration of the knowledge, attitudes, and skills that are most important to a particular task, activity, or role" (Alspach, 1995, p. 162).
- Learning activities are designed to meet regulatory, organizational, departmental, unit, and role requirements of orientation.
- The goals of orientation are clearly defined so all parties involved (orientee, preceptor, educator, supervisor) are clear about their function within and expectations of the orientation process.
- The nursing professional development educator oversees the unit-based orientation process by meeting with the orientee, preceptor, and employee's supervisor to ensure progress is being made toward goals of orientation (Kelly-Thomas, 1998; Alspach, 1995).

PRECEPTOR DEVELOPMENT

- A successful orientation occurs in a precepted, role-modeled environment.
- The roles of a preceptor include that of educator, role-model, and socializer.
  - Educator: Assesses the new hire's learning needs, plans learning activities, implements the teaching plan, and evaluates the orientee's performance
  - Role-model: Demonstrates how the nurse is expected to perform the job
  - Socializer: Makes the orientee feel welcomed and helps her or him to integrate socially and professionally with peer group, unit, and hospital (Alspach, 1995, 2002)
- Preceptor characteristics include desire to teach, positive interpersonal skills, exceptional clinical performance, leadership, and adherence to organizational policy and procedures.

- Collaboratively, the educator and the manager identify employees who exemplify the characteristics needed of preceptors.
- Development of a group of employees who understand the preceptor role and its important function within the organization is the responsibility of the nurse educator.
- Content of a preceptor training program includes:
  - Preceptor roles and responsibilities
  - Reality shock theory
  - Adult education principles
  - Socialization principles
  - Educational process (needs assessment, planning, implementation, and evaluation)
  - Teaching strategies
  - Effective communication and feedback techniques
  - Problem-solving and conflict management
  - Values and cultural impact on the preceptor-preceptee relationship
  - Documentation requirements (Alspach, 1995; Kelly-Thomas, 1998; Speers, Strzyzewski, & Ziolkowski, 2004)
- The preceptor requires support before, during, and after each preceptorship experience from the nursing professional development (NPD) educator and the nurse manager.
  - Before:
    - NPD Educator: Provide a formal, effective preceptor training program and a written preceptor job description
    - Nurse Manager: Provide orientee's resume and self-assessment, interview findings, and compensation in either a financial or career ladder form
  - During:
    - NPD Educator: Maintain close contact to guide the teaching–learning process, address questions, troubleshoot problems, and monitor effectiveness and progress of the program
    - Nurse Manager: Align schedule of preceptor and orientee and ensure staffing is adequate to meet teaching–learning needs
  - After:
    - NPD Educator: Provide regularly scheduled preceptor support groups and continuing education programs on advanced preceptor topics, such as matching teaching and learning styles or creative clinical teaching strategies
    - Nurse Manager: Provide a means of recognition and reward and time away from precepting to prevent burnout or meet preceptor's personal needs (Alspach, 1995)

COMPETENCY MANAGEMENT

- Competence is "a person's capacity to perform his or her job function" (Kelly-Thomas, 1998, p. 74).
- "Competency is the application of knowledge, skills, and behaviors that are needed to fulfill organizational, departmental, and work setting requirements under varied circumstances of the real world" (Wright, 2005, p. 8).

- Competence assessment is a continual process that begins when leaders define the competencies required of a job position and continues with regular validation of an individual's attainment and maintenance of these competencies (Joint Commission Resources, 2007).
- Competencies are broad statements describing general areas of behavior in a particular role and work setting (Alspach, 1995; Joint Commission Resources, 2007) that should:
  - "Describe a general category of behavior
  - Be focused on the learner
  - Be behavioral and measurable
  - Be free from performance conditions
  - Be validated by experts" (Kelly-Thomas, 1998, p. 127)
- Competency statements are written around an organizing framework based on the organization's preference. Example frameworks include nursing diagnoses, nursing process, therapies, nursing practice standards, or medical diagnoses (Alspach, 1995; Kelly-Thomas, 1998).
- Performance criteria represent behaviors that are the essential and observable knowledge, skills, behaviors, and critical thinking of the competency. These behaviors must be performed to validate the competency (Alspach, 1995; Kelly-Thomas, 1998).
- The development of competency statements and performance criteria is a collaborative effort among the nurse educator, nurse manager, clinical nurse specialists, and select nursing staff members (Alspach, 1995).
- Core or initial competencies focus on the knowledge, skills, and abilities needed to perform the job role in the first 6 to 12 months, are grouped into clusters (e.g., communication, care management), and capture the overall job goals (Kelly-Thomas, 1998; Wright, 2005).
- Ongoing competencies reflect the ever-changing nature of the job and the organization's missions and goals (Wright, 2005).
- Ongoing competencies focus on new skills, new products, changes in practice/equipment, and skills that are high-risk, low-volume, or problem-prone (Stafford, 2002; Wright, 2005).
- Various methods may be used to prioritize identified ongoing competencies since the validation process cannot include all competencies. Time, resources, and meaningfulness are considerations for an efficient and cost-effective ongoing competency assessment process.
  - Alspach's (1995) Four Priority Factors
    1. Fatal: High-risk aspects of patient care needs
    2. Fundamental: Essential aspects of effective nursing practice
    3. Frequency: Area of nursing practice that is performed often
    4. Facility/Fixed: Requirement of external accrediting agency or healthcare organization
  - Wright (2005)
    - Is the job aspect in more than one category: new, change, high-risk, problematic?
    - Does the outcome of the competency have an outcome for the patient, customer, or employee?
    - Regarding high-risk job aspects, is it time-sensitive (performance does not allow time to "look it up")?
- The nursing professional development educator works collaboratively with management to identify ongoing competencies and methods for measuring competence.
- The validation process includes many different methods to recognize individual differences in learning styles, demonstration preferences, and experience levels (Wright, 2005). recommends increasing the difficulty or hassle-factor of validation for the learner as time goes on to prevent laggards in the competence assessment process.

- Employees are accountable for ensuring that validation of their competencies occurs; managers are accountable to create systems to support competency assessment (Wright, 2005).
- Assessing competence is done through "processes and programs designed to measure and evaluate the competency of nurses in relation to expected performance standards" (Kelly-Thomas, 1998, p. 26).

INSERVICE

- Inservices are "learning experiences provided in the work setting for the purpose of assisting staff members in performing their assigned functions in that particular agency or institution" (ANA, 2000, p. 24).
- Inservices are a quick response to changes in the work environment (Misko, 2009).
- Learner experiences that take place during work hours in the workplace also are referred to as on-the-job or just-in-time training (Avillion, 2005, 2008).
- Inservice characteristics:
  - "Shorter duration (15 to 60 minutes per session)
  - More informal structure and presentation styles
  - Conducted in or immediately adjacent to the work site
  - Shorter interval between instruction and evaluation of learning
  - May involve faculty who are not hospital staff members
  - Often involve only small group of learners" (Alspach, 1995, p. 237)
- Inservice education methodology depends on the program objectives and learner needs. Methods may include formal lectures, discussions, poster presentations, self-paced learning techniques, and train-the-trainer (Avillion, 2005, 2008).
- Content may include commonly referred to "mandatories": fire safety; back safety; infection control; electrical safety; radiation safety; bloodborne pathogens; and other regulatory, state, and organization requirements.
- The manuals of the accrediting bodies delineate training requirements. Often the organization states the specifics of the requirements within its policies (O'Shea, 2002).
- The nursing professional development educator partners with other departments, for example, infection control and risk management, to identify organizational requirements for inservice content.
- Inservice education also can be incidental learning based on patient situations, medications, and needs. Other informal learning occurs during patient care rounds, discharge planning rounds, and reflection on clinical practice (Alspach, 1995).
- The nursing professional development educator needs to accommodate the learning needs of staff on off shifts. Methodologies that can be employed are self-learning packets, video- or audiotapes with posttests, computer-assisted instruction, designated night/weekend educators, or rotation to nights for educational needs.
- Inservices may be provided by vendor representatives; however, the educator should review the content for appropriateness and ensure it is more than a marketing strategy. Vendor educators can be an excellent source of inservice material and developing collegial relationships with company representatives can be beneficial to the educator and the organization.

- Successful inservices depend on the ability of the educator, availability of equipment, and readiness of the learner. Involve managers to increase attendance at mandatory inservices (Alspach, 1995; Kelly-Thomas, 1998).

CONTINUING EDUCATION

- "The knowledge, skills, or attitudes gained from continuing education activities can be applied regardless of the employer of the activity participant" (ANCC, 2006, p. 7).
- Continuing nursing education (CNE) is viewed as an employee benefit, necessary for continued competence, required for advanced certification, and may or may not be needed for licensure.
- Some states require a specific number of continuing education hours for relicensure; other states may be more prescriptive and require the education be in a certain area such as restraints or forensic evidence collection.
- Some boards of nursing accept CNE activities that have been provided by an ANCC-accredited provider or approved by an ANCC-accredited approver. Others have developed their own mechanisms for approval of CNE activities.
- The nursing professional development curriculum is designed to meet the continuing education (CE) needs of the organization's employees to meet organizational goals and contribute to safe health care (Kelly-Thomas, 1998).
- Continuing education in one's specialty often is required to maintain national certification (ANCC, 2006).
- Continuing education activities fall under the function of a staff development department, but may also be offered by independent agencies, entrepreneurs, or universities (Alspach, 1995).
- The American Nurses Credentialing Center (ANCC) Accreditation Program establishes the standards and criteria for educational programs to be eligible for contact hours for professional nurses.
- The National League of Nursing (NLN) is an Authorized Provider of continuing education by the International Association for Continuing Education and Training. NLN CE programs are limited to those that promote the nursing faculty role (NLN, n.d.).
- In addition to content, the time and cost required to develop and evaluate a CE offering is important to consider when deciding to offer contact hours for an educational activity.
- Continuing nursing education is measured in contact hours calculated from the amount of the educational activity's content that is devoted to transmitting new or transferable knowledge. The minimum time is 30 minutes or 0.5 contact hours (ANCC, 2006).
- CE can be provided in a number of formats:
  - Workshop: Typically a single day for a small group covering in-depth content; may be skill-based with hands-on opportunities
  - Seminar: A small group that exchanges information about a specific topic; requires preparation by the learner
  - Conference: Group process format involving participant discussion related to a single topic area; typically has a coordinator and may last multiple days
  - Course: Comprehensive study of a topic area through a series of learning activities lasting a few days; different than academic courses

- Institute: Formal learning experiences with experts presenting information to participants; often a multiday program
- Symposium: Two or more experts presenting information on a topic, followed by a moderator summary and then a question-and-answer period; can accommodate larger audiences
- Self-study: Varied formats that can include programmed instruction, self-learning packages, reading books or journals, and computer-assisted instruction including online modules, webinars, podcasts, and so on (Alspach, 1995)

CLINICAL AFFILIATIONS

- The nursing professional development educator may be the coordinator for clinical affiliation placements within the healthcare organization.
- Clinical affiliations begin with a memorandum of agreement or contract between the academic institution and the healthcare organization. This contract states the responsibilities of the academic institution, the healthcare organization, the faculty, and the student.
- The nursing professional development educator works with managers of units and areas to identify their willingness and ability to support students within their areas.
- Student learning objectives are obtained from the academic institution to ensure they can be met in the specific clinical areas.
- The nursing professional development educator maintains a schedule of dates and times of clinical group assignment to avert double assignment and unit staff burnout.
- Methodologies to orient faculty to the organization include attendance at nursing or per diem (agency) orientation, self-study packets, and/or computer-assisted instruction, as well as a brief precepted experience on the unit where the faculty member will have students (Duffy, 2001; Stafford, 2009).
- Faculty orientation includes competency in point-of-care or waived testing, medication administration, and documentation.
- Methodologies to orient students include school group orientation by the NPD educator, clinical group orientation by faculty, self-study packets, and/or computer-assisted instruction.
- Other clinical affiliation coordinator duties can include oversight of confidentiality policy and processes for obtaining facility access badges and computer system access.
- Faculty are responsible for supervision and evaluation of clinical nursing student performance; the healthcare institution is responsible for patient care (Duffy, 2001).

REFERENCES

Alspach, J. G. (1995). *The educational process in nursing staff development.* St. Louis, MO: Mosby.

Alspach, J. G. (2002). Preceptor development. In B. E. Puetz & J. W. Aucoin (Eds.) *Conversations in nursing professional development* (pp. 261–272). Pensacola, FL: Pohl Publishing.

American Nurses Association. (2000). *Scope and standards of practice for nursing professional development.* Washington, DC: American Nurses Publishing.

American Nurses Credentialing Center. (2006). *Manual for accreditation as an approver or provider of continuing nursing education: Application manual.* Silver Spring, MD: American Nurses Credentialing Center.

Avillion, A. E. (2005). *Nurse educator manual: Essential skills and guidelines for effective practice.* Marblehead, MA: HCPro.

Avillion, A. E. (2008). *A practical guide to staff development: Tools and techniques for effective education* (2nd ed.). Marblehead, MA: HCPro.

Duffy, M. M. (2001). Arranging clinical affiliations. *Journal for Nurses in Staff Development, 17,* 41–43.

Joint Commission Resources. (2007). *Assessing hospital staff competence* (2nd ed.). Oakbrook Terrace, IL: Joint Commission on Accreditation of Healthcare Organizations.

Kelly-Thomas, K. J. (1998). *Clinical and nursing staff development: Current competence, future focus* (2nd ed.). Philadelphia: Lippincott.

Misko, L. (2009). Implementation of learning activities. In S. L. Bruce (Ed.), *Core curriculum for staff development* (pp. 251–278). Pensacola, FL: National Nursing Staff Development Organization.

National League of Nursing. (n.d.). *Continuing education.* Retrieved from http://www.nln.org/ContinuingEd/index.htm

O'Shea, K. L. (2002). *Staff development nursing secrets.* Philadelphia : Hanley & Belfus.

Speers, A. T., Strzyzewski, N., & Ziolkowski, L. D. (2004). Preceptor preparation: An investment in the future. *Journal for Nurses in Staff Development, 20*(3), 127.

Stafford, R. (2002). Nursing staff development. In B. E. Puetz & J. W. Aucoin (Eds.) *Conversations in nursing professional development* (pp. 35–42). Pensacola, FL: Pohl Publishing.

Wright, D. (2005). *The ultimate guide to competency assessment in health care.* Minneapolis, MN: Creative Health Care Management.

8

Educational Process

BACKGROUND

- The *Scope and Standards of Practice for Nursing Professional Development* (American Nurses Association [ANA], 2000) describes six standards of practice for the nursing professional development educator related to the educational process.
  - Standard I. Assessment: "collects pertinent information related to potential educational needs of the nurse" (p. 12)
  - Standard II. Diagnosis: "analyzes the assessment data to determine the target audience and the learner need" (p. 12)
  - Standard III. Identification of educational outcomes: "identifies the general purpose and educational objectives for each learning activity" (p. 13)
  - Standard IV. Planning: "identifies and collaborates with content experts to develop activities to facilitate learners' achievement of the educational objectives" (p. 13)
  - Standard V. Implementation: "ensures that the planned educational activities are implemented" (p. 14)
  - Standard VI. Evaluation: "conducts a comprehensive evaluation of the educational activity" (p. 15)
- An educational activity is "a planned, organized effort aimed at accomplishing educational objectives" (ANA, 2000, p. 24).

- An educational activity may be in one or more different forms (e.g., lecture, seminar, conference, independent study, simulation, Web-based).
- The American Nurses Credentialing Center (ANCC, 2009) has defined criteria for the needs assessment, planning, implementation, and evaluation of continuing nursing education activities that can be applied to any educational activity. These criteria incorporate adult learning principles as well as professional standards and ethics.

ASSESSMENT

Learning Needs Assessment

- *Learning needs assessment* is a systematic and ongoing process of collecting data to identify gaps between actual and desired knowledge, skills, and/or attitudes (ANA, 2000; Yoder Wise, 1996).
- Needs assessment may be formal or informal.
- Needs assessments provide data that are used to prioritize learning needs, determine the target audience, and distinguish learning needs from systems or performance problems (Avillion, 2008; Cooper, 2002).
- Data are collected from a variety of sources, including:
  - Nurses, other employees, management, administration
  - Healthcare consumers
  - Standards of accrediting organizations
  - Standards of professional organizations
  - Nurse practice acts
  - Legislative rules and regulations
  - Licensure requirements
  - Job descriptions and performance evaluations
  - Professional networks
  - Nursing or healthcare literature
  - Quality improvement data
  - Program evaluation data (Avillion, 2008; Shelton, 2002; Yoder Wise, 1996)
- Data may be collected using various strategies, such as questionnaires, surveys, interviews, focus groups, records, reports, program evaluations, tests, and observations (Kitchie, 2008; Yoder Wise, 1996).
- Data about identified needs are documented in a manner that is retrievable and useful for program planning (ANA, 2000).
- The target audience is the "group for which an educational activity has been designed" (ANA, 2000, p. 26).
- The nursing professional development educator should learn as much as possible about the target audience, including their background, levels of experience, preferred learning styles, motivation to learn, and availability to attend the activity (Bulmer, 2002).
- Steps in conducting a needs assessment:
  - Establish the purpose.
  - Identify the target audience.
  - Decide who will assist with the process.

- Select a method.
- Conduct the needs assessment.
- Analyze and share the results with educators and other stakeholders (Cooper, 2002).

Needs Assessment Strategies

- Questionnaires/Surveys
  - Purpose: To gather information about respondents' opinions rather than objective knowledge or skills.
  - Instruments may be designed with closed-ended questions (e.g., rating scales, multiple choice, Likert scale) or open-ended format (e.g., sentence-completion, completely unstructured) in written or electronic form.
  - Advantages: Can collect information from a large number of respondents in a relatively short time; most learners are familiar with this type of format; forms can be completed anonymously, encouraging honest opinions; if closed-ended questions are used, data are easily tabulated and analyzed.
  - Disadvantages: Possibility of low response rate; learners may not understand items; no opportunity to clarify vague or ambiguous items or responses; open-ended questions may be time-consuming to analyze (Kitchie, 2008; Yoder Wise, 1996).
- Interviews
  - Purpose: To provide for in-depth discussion of learning needs and areas of concern.
  - Interviews may be structured (specific sequence of direct, focused questions) or unstructured (general question with follow-up).
  - Advantages: More in-depth, thorough responses, especially if rapport established; responses can be clarified with follow-up questions.
  - Disadvantages: Information subjectively interpreted by the interviewer; interviewees may provide responses that they think the interviewer wants to hear; responses, especially in unstructured interview, may be difficult to objectively analyze (Kitchie, 2008; Yoder Wise, 1996).
- Focus Groups
  - Purpose: To provide for in-depth discussion about a specific learning need or topic.
  - A focus group consists of 4 to 12 potential learners who participate in a 60- to 90-minute discussion.
  - A facilitator leads the discussion by asking open-ended questions that encourage dialogue.
  - An observer is present to take notes and/or record the discussion with permission of the participants.
  - Advantages: Source of rich qualitative data about specific learning needs; conveys sense of value for learners' ideas and opinions.
  - Disadvantages: Participants may feel some reluctance to honestly express ideas; may be time-consuming to analyze (Cooper, 2002; Kitchie, 2008; Yoder Wise, 1996).
- Records/Reports
  - Purpose: To gather information from existing data sources that may illustrate learning needs.
  - Examples of reports that are commonly used to assess learning needs include quality improvement reports and audits, patient record audits, infection control reports, event reports, annual reports, and patient surveys.
  - Records that provide needs assessment data may include program evaluation summaries, meeting minutes, position descriptions, and performance appraisals.

- Advantages: Process and tools are already in place and readily accessible; identified learning needs relate to organizational priorities.
  - Disadvantages: Findings may reflect organizational system needs rather than individual learning needs; may be time-consuming to analyze (Cooper, 2002; Yoder Wise, 1996).
- Tests
  - Purpose: To assess knowledge and skill levels on a specific topic to identify gaps and tailor teaching to meet learning needs.
  - Testing is complex. The test developer must use a test blueprint and consider validity, reliability, pilot testing, and criterion or norm-referenced grading. (See Chapter 11 for more information on test development.)
  - Advantages: Findings helpful to tailor educational plan to specific audience.
  - Disadvantages: Data may reflect problems with test-taking ability rather than learning needs; time-consuming to develop a valid and reliable testing tool (Kitchie, 2008; Yoder Wise, 1996).
- Observations
  - Purpose: To validate data from other sources and determine discrepancies between stated behavior and actual behavior.
  - Observations may be planned or incidental.
  - Specific standards must be used to observe behavior, and observed behaviors must be documented using a checklist or other form of documentation.
  - If multiple observers are involved, interrater reliability must be determined.
  - Advantages: Provide information about actual values and performance rather than reported values and performance; excellent source of information about needs related to performance of skills.
  - Disadvantages: Person being observed may alter behaviors if he or she knows observation is occurring; time-consuming for observer (Yoder Wise, 1996).
- When possible, needs assessment data should be validated using more than one data collection method (e.g., gap identified in infection control data confirmed through staff survey; Shelton, 2002).
- The nursing professional development educator objectively analyzes data from multiple sources (e.g., survey, event report, administrative mandate) to determine learning needs before developing an educational plan.
- The nursing professional development educator involves key stakeholders in prioritizing learning needs based on factors such as organizational goals, available financial and staff resources, and the significance of the need to patient care (Cooper, 2002; Shelton, 2002).

PLANNING

General Principles

- The educational planning process involves development of a clear purpose or goal statement, measurable objectives that are appropriate for the target audience, content, teaching methods, and evaluation strategies.
- A *purpose statement*, often referred to as a learning goal, describes the target audience and intended outcome for an educational activity (ANA, 2000).

- *Behavioral objectives* are based on identified learning needs.
- Behavioral objectives clearly state the learner outcomes of an educational activity in specific and measurable terms (Bastable & Doody, 2008).
- Content for an educational activity is congruent with the activity's purpose and educational objectives.
- Teaching and learning strategies are congruent with the activity's objectives and content.
- The nursing professional development educator defines a clear method to evaluate an educational activity and determine whether the educational objectives were met (ANCC, 2009).

Writing Behavioral Objectives

- The principles of adult learning are incorporated in the development of educational objectives.
- Objectives are written in behavioral terms appropriate to the target audience and specifically identify what the learner must accomplish.
- Each objective contains only one expected behavior.
- Behavioral objectives describe learner outcomes in the cognitive, psychomotor, and/or affective domains of learning (see Chapter 3 for information on the domains of learning).
- Objectives must contain an action verb that explicitly identifies in observable and measurable terms what the learner must do to successfully complete the learning activity.
- Well-written objectives include four components that can be represented by the acronym ABCD:
  - **Audience:** identifies the learner as the focus (who)
  - **Behavior:** action that the learner will be able to do to demonstrate that learning has occurred (what)
  - **Condition:** refers to the circumstances under which the learner is expected to perform the actions (how)
  - **Degree of attainment:** describes the standard (e.g., accuracy, timing, amount) to which actions must be done to be acceptable (how well; Bastable & Doody, 2008; Bruce, 2002).
- Sample objectives for each domain of learning
  - Cognitive: After completing a self-learning module (C), the learner (A) is able to explain (B) the action of three chemotherapeutic agents (D) used in the treatment of breast cancer.
  - Psychomotor: Given a selection of dressing supplies (C), the learner (A) is able to demonstrate (B) a sterile dressing change following the institutional guideline (D).
  - Affective: Following a facilitated group discussion (C), the learner (A) is able to implement (B) three strategies for overcoming barriers to caring for patients from other cultures (D).

Content Determination

- *Content* is the "subject matter of the educational activity that relates to the educational objectives" (ANA, 2000, p. 23).
- Content is individualized to the target audience, according to the participants' basic education, advanced education, experience, and preferred learning style.
- The nursing professional development educator collaborates with members of the target audience and content experts to develop content for an educational activity (ANCC, 2009).
- Content is developed in a cost-efficient manner using available resources.

- Content is organized in a logical and meaningful sequence, congruent with the activity's learning objectives.
- Content may be structured to present general concepts followed by specific examples, simple to complex, theoretical principles to practical application, chronological order, or some other logical flow of information (DeYoung, 2009; Leroux & Cody, 1996).

Selection of Faculty and Content Experts

- Faculty and content experts must have credible experience and expertise in the content to be presented.
- Faculty must have knowledge of the educational process, including principles of adult learning and learning styles.
- Faculty must use an informative, engaging presentation style that encourages participation, addresses participant questions, and incorporates techniques that are appropriate to the objectives.
- Faculty must be comfortable presenting content using the teaching format identified (e.g., distance learning, videotape).
- Content experts must use current expertise and an evidence-based approach to develop content for independent study modules and other types of learner-paced activities.
- Faculty and content experts may be identified from within or external to the organization (Bulmer, 2002).
- Those from within the organization:
  - Know the organizational culture, goals, and objectives
  - Know and are known to the target audience
  - May be expected to present educational activities as part of their role
  - May not be able to bring unique or external perspective to the audience
- Those external to the organization:
  - Bring external perspective to an educational activity
  - May be perceived as more prestigious than internal presenters
  - Require a contract or letter of agreement outlining needs and expenses
  - May be unaware of organizational culture, goals, and objectives

Selection of Teaching Strategies

- *Teaching strategies* are "instructional methods and techniques that are in accord with principles of adult learning" (ANCC, 2009, p. 76).
- A variety of teaching strategies may be necessary to promote learning in adults who have different backgrounds, experience, and learning style preferences (O'Shea, 2002).
- The nursing professional development educator selects teaching strategies after considering several factors, including:
  - Adult learning principles
  - Audience characteristics (e.g., group size, diversity, level of expertise)
  - Educator's expertise and preferences for teaching strategies
  - Learning objectives
  - Complexity of content

- Cost-effectiveness
- Setting for educational activity
- Time
- Available resources (e.g., technology aids, materials, manikins; Fitzgerald, 2008)
- Clark (2008) identified four qualities of teaching methods to consider when teaching.
  1. Fidelity means that the strategy closely aligns in realism to the actual situation.
  2. Cost refers to the expense of a teaching strategy.
  3. Safety can be applied to the patient (e.g., risk of harm) or the learner (e.g., negative experience).
  4. Completeness means that the strategy provides practice opportunities that may not be immediately available in the real world.

Description of Teaching Strategies

- Lecture
  - Structured method in which the presenter uses a prepared oral presentation to give new information to groups of learners
  - Useful when a large amount of information must be presented to large groups
  - Limited flexibility in scheduling or delivery of content
  - More effective if opportunities for interaction and feedback are incorporated through a combination of lecture with small group discussion, group exercises, question-and-answer sessions, audiovisual aids, or other interactive strategies (Aucoin, 1998; Fitzgerald, 2008; Rowles & Russo, 2009)
- Group discussion
  - Method of teaching whereby learners exchange information and opinions with one another and the presenter
  - Useful for problem-solving, exploring attitudes, sharing information, and critique of concepts when participants have some knowledge of topic
  - May want to incorporate visuals or hands-on activities to involve more than the auditory sense
  - Allows for clarification of information, response to questions, and discussion of concerns
  - Less faculty control and structure (Fitzgerald, 2008; Gianella, 1996)
- Demonstration
  - Most frequently used for psychomotor skills
  - Engages the learner through stimulation of visual, auditory, and tactile senses
  - Often used in combination with return demonstration to validate learner achievement of objectives
  - Requires adequate time, ample equipment, and small group size to provide opportunity for practice and supervision (Fitzgerald, 2008; Rowles & Russo, 2009)
- Role play
  - Experiential learning method in which learners participate in a dramatization of a real work situation or a case study
  - Often used to achieve objectives in the affective domain but may be used for cognitive and psychomotor domain objectives
  - Learners may volunteer or be assigned to a defined role in the situation
  - Useful to enhance problem-solving and critical thinking skills
  - Best done in small groups in a nonthreatening environment to encourage participation and active involvement

- Debriefing occurs at the conclusion of the dramatization (Clark, 2008; Fitzgerald, 2008; O'Shea, 2002)
- Simulation
  - Experiential learning method in which a clinical situation is replicated in accuracy and detail in a safe environment
  - Used to teach cognitive, psychomotor, and affective domains
  - May be done using written scenarios, videotape, models, actors, peers, and/or high-fidelity manikins
  - Allows for realistic learner involvement in managing or responding to a clinical situation as an individual or as a member of a team
  - Useful when situation occurs infrequently in the clinical setting or when learning in the actual work setting may compromise patient safety or is ethically or legally questionable
  - Debriefing occurs at the conclusion of the simulation (Fitzgerald, 2008; Gianella, 1996)
- Gaming
  - Experiential learning method in which learners apply knowledge and skills as they participate in a structured, competitive activity
  - Used primarily for cognitive domain but may be used to supplement skills and behavior in psychomotor and affective domains
  - Effective for review or reinforcement of content
  - May be designed for individual or team use
  - May be fun but also needs to contribute to achievement of learning objectives
  - Competitive environment may be threatening to some learners
  - Debriefing occurs at the conclusion of the game to highlight key concepts (Fitzgerald, 2008; Gianella, 1996; O'Shea, 2002; Rowles & Russo, 2009)
- Posters
  - Visual representation of concepts to convey information
  - Colorful, visually stimulating format to convey detailed information in a concise way
  - Allows learner to review information at a comfortable pace
  - Useful to share procedural or process information or visual content (Aucoin, 1998; Rowles & Russo, 2009)
- Self-learning modules
  - Packets of materials designed for independent study of a specific topic at the learner's pace
  - Faculty serves as a facilitator and resource to the learner
  - Used primarily for learning in the cognitive domain and the psychomotor domain if learning objectives include application to practice
  - Alternative to traditional methods when learners are not readily able to leave the work unit for a class
  - Effective for self-directed learners who are self-disciplined to complete the required work in a timely manner
  - May include various learning media such as articles, handouts, Web pages, audiovisuals, and equipment displays (Aucoin, 1998; Fitzgerald, 2008; Gianella, 1996; O'Shea, 2002)
- Computer-assisted instruction
  - Delivery of educational content electronically
  - Used primarily to promote learning in the cognitive domain
  - May be in the form of computer or Web-based presentations, tutorials, drill and practice, simulations, or testing
  - Requires funding to develop or purchase

- Limited opportunity for interaction with other learners or educator unless Web-based format
- Must have adequate technological knowledge or support to implement and use effectively (Bowman, 2002; Clark, 2008; DeYoung, 2009; Hainsworth, 2008)
- Case studies/grand rounds
  - Analysis and application of theoretical content to a reality-based situation
  - Used effectively to reinforce theoretical content by presenting complex situations requiring application of content using problem-solving and critical thinking
  - Well-designed case study is key to successful achievement of learning objectives
  - Most effective in an open, nonthreatening, interactive learning environment
  - Link between theoretical and practical content encourages retention of important information (Aucoin, 1998; Rowles & Russo, 2009)
- Learning contract
  - Individualized written or verbal agreement between faculty and student that describes what the learner must do to achieve learning objectives, what resources faculty provides, and criteria that will be used to determine success
  - Identifies behavioral objectives to be achieved, instructional strategies and resources, method of evaluation of objective achievement, and target dates for completion
  - Empowers the learner because contract development emphasizes self-direction and negotiation for learning activities and outcomes
  - Actively involves the learner at all stages of the educational process from learning needs assessment through evaluation (Bastable & Doody, 2008; DeYoung, 2009)
- Others
  - Many other strategies or variations of those listed above are available.
  - Some of these include debate, role-modeling, storytelling, online forum, and videoconference

IMPLEMENTATION

General Principles

- According to Standard V of the *Scope and Standards of Practice for Nursing Professional Development* (ANA, 2000), "the nursing professional development educator ensures that the planned educational activities are implemented ... in a timely and appropriate manner."
- In addition, in the same document Standard VIII of Professional Performance states "the nursing professional development educator considers factors related to safety, effectiveness, and cost in planning, delivering, and managing nursing professional development activities (ANA, 2000, p. 21).

See Chapter 9 for information pertaining to design and delivery skills.

EVALUATION

Outcomes

- An *outcome* is the "end result of a learning activity measured by written evaluation or change in practice" (ANA, 2000, p. 25).
- Outcomes usually involve a change in knowledge, competence, practice, or patient care.
- Learning outcomes are identified by the behavioral objectives and are consistent with the educational activity's purpose and teaching strategies.
- The evaluation process measures the achievement of learning outcomes in relation to the intended learning outcomes (Kirkpatrick & DeWitt, 2009; Webb, 2002).

See Chapter 11 for a discussion of types and models of evaluation as well as uses of evaluative data.

REFERENCES

Alspach, J. G. (1995). *The educational process in nursing staff development.* St. Louis, MO: Mosby.

American Nurses Association. (2000). *Scope and standards of practice for nursing professional development.* Washington, DC: American Nurses Publishing.

American Nurses Credentialing Center. (2009). *Application manual: Accreditation program.* Silver Spring, MD: American Nurses Credentialing Center.

Aucoin, J. W. (1998). Program planning: Solving the problem. In K. J. Kelly-Thomas, *Clinical and nursing staff development: Current competence, future focus* (2nd. ed., pp. 213–239). Philadelphia: Lippincott.

Avillion, A. E. (2008). *A practical guide to staff development: Evidence-based tools and techniques for effective education* (2nd ed.). Marblehead, MA: HC Pro.

Bastable, S. B., & Doody, J. A. (2008). Behavioral objectives. In S. B. Bastable (Ed.), *Nurse as educator: Principles of teaching and learning for nursing practice* (3rd ed., pp. 383–427). Boston: Jones & Bartlett.

Bowman, K. R. (2002). Using computers in education. In K. L. O'Shea, *Staff development nursing secrets* (pp. 139–147). Philadelphia: Hanley & Belfus.

Bruce, S. L. (2002). Writing objectives. In B. E. Puetz & J. W. Aucoin (Eds.), *Conversations in nursing professional development* (pp. 139–150). Pensacola, FL: Pohl Publishing.

Bulmer, J. M. (2002). Program planning. In K. L. O'Shea, *Staff development nursing secrets* (pp. 79–93). Philadelphia: Hanley & Belfus.

Clark, C. C. (2008). *Classroom skills for nurse educators.* Sudbury, MA: Jones & Bartlett

Cooper, D. C. (2002). Needs assessment. In K. L. O'Shea. *Staff development nursing secrets* (pp. 65–78). Philadelphia: Hanley & Belfus.

DeYoung, S. (2009). *Teaching strategies for nurse educators* (2nd ed.). Upper Saddle River, NJ: Prentice Hall.

Fitzgerald, K. (2008). Instructional methods and settings. In S. B. Bastable (Ed.), *Nurse as educator: Principles of teaching and learning for nursing practice* (3rd ed., pp. 429–471). Boston: Jones & Bartlett.

Gianella, A. (1996). Effective teaching and learning strategies for adults. In R. S. Abruzzese (Ed.), *Nursing staff development: Strategies for success* (2nd ed., pp. 223–241). St. Louis, MO: Mosby.

Hainsworth, D. S. (2008). Instructional materials. In S. B. Bastable (Ed.), *Nurse as educator: Principles of teaching and learning for nursing practice* (3rd ed., pp. 473–514). Boston: Jones & Bartlett.

Kirkpatrick, J. M., & DeWitt, D. A. (2009). Strategies for assessing/evaluating learning outcomes. In D. M. Billings & J. A. Halstead (Eds.), *Teaching in nursing: A guide for faculty* (3rd ed., pp. 409–428). St. Louis, MO: Saunders.

Kitchie, S. (2008). Determinants of learning. In S. B. Bastable (Ed.), *Nurse as educator: Principles of teaching and learning for nursing practice* (3rd ed., pp. 93–145). Boston: Jones & Bartlett.

Leroux, D. S., & Cody, B. (1996). Curriculum planning and development. In R. S. Abruzzese (Ed.), *Nursing staff development: Strategies for success.* (2nd ed., pp. 209–222). St. Louis, MO: Mosby.

O'Shea, K. L. (2002). *Staff development nursing secrets.* Philadelphia: Hanley & Belfus.

Rowles, C. J., & Russo, B. L. (2009). Strategies to promote critical thinking and active learning. In D. M. Billings & J. A. Halstead (Eds.), *Teaching in nursing: A guide for faculty* (3rd ed., pp. 238–261). St. Louis, MO: Saunders.

Shelton, D. P. (2002). Assessing learning needs. In B. E. Puetz & J. W. Aucoin (Eds.), *Conversations in nursing professional development* (pp. 133–137). Pensacola, FL: Pohl Publishing.

Webb, D. G. (2002). Evaluating. In B. E. Puetz & J. W. Aucoin (Eds.), *Conversations in nursing professional development* (pp. 177–183). Pensacola, FL: Pohl Publishing.

Yoder Wise, P. S. (1996). Learning needs assessment. In R. S. Abruzzese (Ed.), *Nursing staff development: Strategies for success* (2nd ed., pp.188–207). St. Louis, MO: Mosby.

9

Design and Delivery Skills

PRESENTATION SKILLS

Preparation

- Know the audience; address their needs.
- Select content based on learning objectives.
- Define the purpose; the lecture method is not appropriate for all content.
- Organize the information: simple to complex, according to issues, or according to a timeline; tell them what you are going to tell them, tell them, tell them what you told them.
- Use an outline to assist with a logical presentation with clear connections.
- Presentation components:
  - Introduction that captures audience's attention
  - Three to five core messages in the body of the talk
  - Conclusion that focuses on a call to action, an inspiration, or a summary
- Content is current and evidence-based
- Anticipate audience questions, have answers prepared or incorporated into content
- Practice with one or several people who will give you constructive feedback (Paterson, 2002; Vollman, 2005).

Delivery

- Avoid alcohol and difficult-to-digest foods the night before a presentation.
- A prespeech warm-up can consist of affirming, breathing, and composing oneself.
- Start with a powerful introduction to capture attention within the first 90 seconds.
- Maintain eye contact throughout the presentation.
- Strengthen message using "hooks" (e.g., humor, analogies, personal experiences).
- Use body language and voice to emphasize points.
- Change from lecture to another teaching strategy (e.g., asking audience to share, using audio/video clips) every 10 to 20 minutes to hold audience attention.
- Do not read verbatim from notes.
- Do not turn back to audience to read from slides.
- Be prepared to extract a section if low on time or add a section if there is time left.
- Use the question-and-answer period to reinforce key messages (Paterson, 2002; Vollman, 2005).

Motivating Participants and Keeping Their Attention

- Create a positive and interesting environment for learners to motivate themselves.
- Recognize the value of the learners.
- Involve learners in the educational process.
- Gain learners' commitment by asking them what they want to gain in the class.
- Vary the teaching methods every 10 to 20 minutes.
- Use activities that require physical movement to teach or reinforce the message (Deck, 2002).
- Use the Attention, Relevance, Confidence, and Satisfaction (ARCS) Model of Motivational Design:
  - Sustain listeners' interest and curiosity (attention)
  - Make presentation relevant and satisfying (relevance)
  - Instill confidence; success encourages the learner to proceed (confidence)
  - Leave satisfied after a learning goal has been achieved (satisfaction) (Paterson, 2002)

Tips to Help Learning

- Content makes sense.
- Content is related to the role of the learner.
- Content can be realistically applied.
- Content is presented in manageable increments.
- The presenter has credibility.
- The presentation is lively.
- Potential obstacles to implementation are addressed.
- Opportunities exist for implementation of new or reinforced knowledge and skills.
- Opportunities exist for reflection on the implementation process.
- The learner is continually challenged to grow (Dickerson, 2003).

IMAGES AND HANDOUTS

Images

- Need to be visible by participants
- Must add to content, not merely be decorative
- Make the message easier for the learner
- Focus participant attention to one place
- Avoid images and graphics that are not related to the content
- Consider copyright issues related to images (see Chapter 4 for discussion of copyright considerations).

Handouts

- Used for participant to follow along; however, allows participant to also look ahead.
- Include a content outline of the major concepts.
- Keep to a maximum of 10 pages.
- Can include the "nice to know" that is not covered due to time limitations.
- Include graphs, charts, etc., from visuals.
- Handouts must be clear, clean copies and typed, never handwritten.
- When handouts are produced from electronic slides (i.e., PowerPoint), ensure all content can be read in the smaller format.
- Do not reproduce copyrighted material without written permission from the copyright holder.
- Handouts may be enhanced with illustrations, but do not overwhelm the reader with too much color or "action."
- Preprinted educational material is available from third parties (Avillion, 2008).

Flip Charts

- Flip charts can be especially useful for group activities, focus groups, and problem-solving activities.
- Limit information on each page to avoid confusion.
- Use dark colors and print in capital letters to enhance readability.
- Flip-chart content can be prepared ahead or added during the presentation.
- Completed pages can be posted in the room for later reference.
- Flip-chart paper is available plain, with lines or grids, and may have removable adhesive.
- Flip charts are not feasible for large audiences due to size limitation (Alspach, 1995; Misko, 2009).

Electronic Slides

- Present one main concept on each slide.
- Include information on slides to support and reinforce key concepts.
- Use key words and phrases, not sentences.

- Use a maximum of six lines per slide and six words per line.
- Avoid using multicolored backgrounds, which compete with written words and make them hard to distinguish.
- The greater the contrast between text and background color, the easier to see for participant,
- A lighter background with dark text may be more visible in a well-lit room, while lighter text on a dark background works better in a dimly lit room.
- Do not use more than two different font styles.
- Sans serif fonts (e.g., Arial) are easier for the eye to see on a computer or projection screen; serif fonts (e.g., Times New Roman) are easier for the eye to follow on paper where lines of text are longer.
- The font size should be at least 24 point; check projection in the room for visibility.
- Avoid all capitals, italics, and red font color because these are difficult for the eye to read. For emphasis use bold, shadowing, different font color, or place text within a shape (e.g., oval, box).
- Keep bullets and slide transitions consistent throughout presentation.
- Do not overwhelm the viewer with moving objects and slide animation.
- Use sound effects, music, etc., to enhance, not compete with, written concepts.
- Include graphs, charts, and demographics as part of the handout in addition to including them in the computer presentation.
- Use visuals in addition to text whenever possible.
- When embedding video clips or Internet links, verify before the presentation that they work with the set-up to be used.
- While electronic slides load faster when on the computer's hard drive, always bring a back-up copy.
- Electronic slides are portable and easily updated, reorganized, and stored (Paradi, 2003; Wilkinson, 2002).

Flyers

- Flyers are typically used to alert internal customers of upcoming educational activities.
- Information to include on flyers: name of program, dates, times, location, and target audience.
- Include the purpose of the program, the speaker, and if contact hours are available to peek interest of potential attendees.
- Lay information out clearly, providing enough white space for ease of readability.
- Use of attractive color(s) is eye-catching.
- Proofread to avoid errors, especially in date, time, and location (Bodin, 2009).

Reports

- The nursing professional development educator frequently compiles reports for results of needs assessments, educational program activities, and evaluation summaries.
- Reports are to be timely, collated for confidentiality and professional presentation.
- Reports are laid out in a logical fashion.
- Depending on the length, a table of contents may be helpful.
- Include graphic data representation for illustration and understanding.
- Proofread for errors and accuracy of data.
- Disseminate report to appropriate stakeholders (Warren, 2009).

USE OF TECHNOLOGY

- Technology addresses adult learning principles by meeting individual learning styles, providing interactivity, and offering self-paced learning.
- Types of technology that can be used in the learning environment include tele- and videoconferencing, webinars, computer-based training, Internet, and high-fidelity simulators.
- The use of these modalities is classified as e-learning (Bowman, 2002).
- Choose a technology that enhances the content; the goal is to make it easier for the learner to remember the message.
- When using technology, ensure visual and audio will function in the presentation room.
- Verify that software versions are compatible between electronic file and computer.
- Know how to troubleshoot technology or whom to contact for timely assistance.
- The nursing professional development educator facilitates the learner's adaptation to new technology by providing instruction and practice with the technology, demonstrating the technology's relationship to improved patient care, and providing emotional support.
- The nursing professional development educator provides assistance with computer literacy.
- E-learning can reduce the time the nurse educator spends providing repetitive training and can augment knowledge acquisition so time in the classroom can be spent on application (Bowman, 2002).
- Computer-based training (CBT) is typically the first step into the use of technology. CBT can be purchased from vendors or developed in-house if the organization has the resources.
- Vendors who supply CBT also may provide learning management systems (LMS). An LMS may be limited to attendance records or provide a level of sophistication that allows course registration, rosters, name tags, grade sheets, and reports can be created (Bowman, 2002).
- Limitations to the use of technology include:
  - High cost
  - Availability of computer resources
  - Computer literacy of learner and instructor
  - Technology failure
  - Content not appropriate for technology
- Benefits to the use of technology include:
  - Rapid knowledge dissemination
  - Decrease in face-to-face training time
  - Engage participants with different learning styles
  - Flexibility with asynchronous learning (DiMauro, 2002; Gloe, 2002; Hartwell, 2009).

TEST CONSTRUCTION

- Tests are commonly used to evaluate the cognitive domain, although a skill demonstration test can be used to evaluate the psychomotor domain.
- Tests need to be valid and reliable to ensure they are measuring the desired outcome.
- A valid test measures what it is expected to measure.

- Reliability means the test consistently yields the same, or nearly the same, score for an individual taking the test several times during a span in which the trait being measured is not expected to change.
- The length of a test is determined by the amount of time that can be devoted to testing.
- Typically, a learner is given one minute for each multiple choice question. Alternative item types may require longer times for responses (Haladyna, 1999; Kubisyn & Borich, 2000; Oermann & Gaberson, 2006).

Validity

- Content validity is assessed by comparing test items to learning objectives to see if they match. A test blueprint assists with this task.
- A test blueprint is a grid with the objectives written down the first column and the cognitive domain levels (knowledge, comprehension, application, etc.) in ascending order along the top row.
- The total number of test questions is divided among the objectives according to importance and each objective's cognitive domain level. The higher the cognitive level, the more questions can be asked to that objective.
- Questions are developed at the objective's domain level and lower. For example, if an objective is at the application level, the questions pertaining to that level are written at the application level and may include questions at the knowledge and comprehension level.
- The grid is filled in with the numbers of questions for each objective in each domain.
- The questions are then reviewed according to the test blueprint to ensure the questions address the objectives at the levels indicated.
- Writing test items at different cognitive levels is a learned skill and develops with practice.
- When using a test bank, ensure the questions align with content and domain level of the objectives (Haladyna, 1999; Kubisyn & Borich, 2000; Oermann & Gaberson, 2006).

Reliability

- Reliability is best determined when a test is designed to measure a single basic concept.
- Reliability is affected by group variability, the number of test items, and the difficulty of test items.
- "All tests are imperfect and are subject to error" (Kubisyn & Borich, 2000, p. 321). Therefore, it is important for the nursing professional development educator to take steps to increase the accuracy and decrease the error of tests.
- These steps include:
  - Have distractors of the multiple choice items be plausible to the uninformed
  - Ensure that no test item is dependent on the learner's response to another question
  - Remove ambiguous questions
  - Write the test at an appropriate reading level
  - Have clear, specific, written directions for completing the test
  - Verify the test answer key is correct (Haladyna, 1999; Kubisyn & Borich, 2000; Oermann & Gaberson, 2006)

Difficulty Level

- The purpose of the test determines the difficulty level of test items even when items are written at higher cognitive levels.
- If the purpose is to verify the learner has "gotten" the message, such as with mandatory training, then the goal is 100% for passing. In other words, 100% of the people responding to the question answer it correctly.
- If the purpose is to ensure the learner can function in a specific unit at a specific level, such as for a critical care course, then the goal may be 80% for passing. In other words, 80% of the people responding to the question answer it correctly.
- Review questions to determine that the distractors are plausible and not obviously incorrect answers.
- If a large percentage of learners selects the incorrect answer, determine if the item was keyed wrong, there was an error in the question, or the teaching did not address the learning need (Haladyna, 1999; Kubisyn & Borich, 2000).

REFERENCES

Alspach, J. G. (1995). *The educational process in nursing staff development.* St. Louis, MO: Mosby.

Avillion, A. E. (2008). *A practical guide to staff development: Evidence-based tools and techniques for effective education* (2nd ed.). Marblehead, MA: HCPro.

Bodin, S. (2009). Marketing educational activities. In S. L. Bruce (Ed.), *Core curriculum for staff development* (3rd ed., pp. 347–360). Pensacola, FL: National Nursing Staff Development Organization.

Bowman, K. R. (2002). Using computers in education. In K. L. O'Shea, *Staff development nursing secrets* (pp. 139–147). Philadelphia: Hanley & Belfus.

Deck, M. L. (2002). Educator. In B. E. Puetz & J. W. Aucoin (Eds.), *Conversations in nursing professional development* (pp. 61–67). Pensacola, FL: Pohl Publishing.

Dickerson, P. S. (2003). Ten tips to help learning. *Journal of Nurses in Staff Development, 19,* 244–250.

DiMauro, N. M. (2002). Integrating technology choices into practice. In B. E. Puetz & J. W. Aucoin (Eds.), *Conversations in nursing professional development* (pp. 287–302). Pensacola, FL: Pohl Publishing.

Gloe, D. (2002). Teaching about computer use. In B. E. Puetz & J. W. Aucoin (Eds.), *Conversations in nursing professional development* (pp. 303–312). Pensacola, FL: Pohl Publishing.

Haladyna, T. M. (1999). *Developing and validating multiple-choice test items* (2nd ed.). Mahwah, NJ: Lawrence Erlbaum Associates.

Hartwell, S. (2009). Technology and staff development. In S. L. Bruce (Ed.), *Core curriculum for staff development* (3rd ed., pp. 279–295). Pensacola, FL: National Nursing Staff Development Organization.

Kubisyn, T., & Borich, G. (2000). *Educational testing and measurement: Classroom application and practice* (6th ed.). New York, NY: John Wiley & Sons.

Misko, L. (2009). Implementation of learning activities. In S. L. Bruce (Ed.), *Core curriculum for staff development* (3rd ed., pp. 251–278). Pensacola, FL: National Nursing Staff Development Organization.

Oermann, M. H., & Gaberson, K. B. (2006). *Evaluation and testing in nursing education* (2nd ed.). New York: Springer Publishing.

Paradi, D. (2003). *Ten secrets for using PowerPoint effectively.* Retrieved from http://www.thinkoutsidetheslide.com/articles/ten_secrets_for_using_powerpoint.htm

Paterson, B. L. (2002). Presentation skills. In K. L. O'Shea, *Staff development nursing secrets* (pp. 123–129). Philadelphia: Hanley & Belfus.

Vollman, K. M. (2005). Enhancing presentation skills for the advanced practice nurse: Strategies for success. *AACN Clinical Issues, 16,* 67–77.

Warren, J. (2009). Program evaluation/return on investment. In S. L. Bruce (Ed.), *Core curriculum for staff development* (3rd ed., pp. 297–320). Pensacola, FL: National Nursing Staff Development Organization.

Wilkinson, C. S. (2002). Implementing. In B. E. Puetz, & J. W. Aucoin (Eds.), *Conversations in nursing professional development* (pp. 157–170). Pensacola, FL: Pohl Publishing.

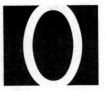

Marketing and Management of Educational Activities

MARKETING EDUCATIONAL ACTIVITIES

Marketing

- *Marketing* is the "creation of services or products to meet customers' needs" (Rodriguez, 1996).
- "Marketing and promotional materials must accurately reflect all aspects of the educational activity" (American Nurses Association [ANA], 2000).
- *Internal marketing* is marketing that is directed to learners and their managers within one's own place of employment (Aucoin, 1998b).
- *External marketing* is marketing that is directed to prospective learners outside the organization (Aucoin, 1998b).
- The goal of marketing in nursing professional development is to promote educational products and services that will support the organization's strategic goals and values, meet the learning needs identified by staff, and adhere to criteria of accrediting bodies.
- The components of marketing are:
  - Completion of marketing analysis
  - Development of a marketing plan
  - Implementation of a marketing plan
  - Management of the overall process (Alspach, 1995)

- A market analysis for nursing professional development includes:
  - Educational needs assessment
  - Characteristics of the target audience
  - Assessment of inconsistencies in practice in the patient care environment
  - Understanding of trends in health care, nursing practice, social and demographic environment
  - Examination of fiscal, legislative, regulatory, and accreditation environment and factors
  - Understanding of the mission, strategic goals, and objectives of the organization
  - Extent of resources (Alspach, 1995; Rodriguez, 1996)

The Five "P's" of a Marketing Plan

- *Product* refers to the items (tangible) or services (intangible) that are offered to customers.
  - Nursing professional development products may include classes, workshops, self-directed learning modules, audiovisual programs, and computer-based instruction.
  - Both learners and decision-makers must desire the product(s).
  - The nursing professional development educator is responsible for assuring the quality of product objectives, content, and teaching strategies, regardless of whether the source is internal or external to the organization (Rodriguez, 1996).
- *Place* is the location of the educational activity.
  - Considerations in selecting an internal location include comfort, size, adequate lighting and ventilation, acoustic quality, visibility of presenter and audiovisuals, and accessibility.
  - Additional considerations in selecting an external location include cost, parking availability, appropriateness of setting, adjacent facilities, and security.
  - Internal locations may be a conference room or classroom on or off a work unit, a skills lab, lecture hall, computer lab, or simulation center.
  - External locations may be a conference or convention center, public meeting space, or hotel.
- *Price* refers to the cost of attendance at the educational activity.
  - The pricing objective may be to generate a profit, break even, or absorb the loss.
  - The organization's mission and policies as well as an internal versus external marketing focus may influence the pricing objective (e.g., employees attend free).
  - Price is determined by the pricing objective, market considerations, and total budget.
  - If a registration fee is assessed, it should be high enough to reflect that the program has educational value but not so high that it is overpriced and discourages attendance (Aucoin, 1998b).
- *Promotion* is the action taken to communicate information about an educational activity to the target audience in a timely manner.
  - Promotion may be accomplished through brochures, fliers, e-mails, notices in newsletters or on bulletin boards, slogans, logos, printed or electronic catalogs, word of mouth, electronic calendars or notices, mailings, social networking sites, and public announcements.
  - The availability of fiscal, material, and human resources and the scope and size of the target audience may influence the selection of promotion strategies (Alspach, 1995).
- *Participants* are the identified members of the target audience for the educational activity.
  - Professional and personal characteristics of the target audience should be considered in the marketing plan.

- Information gathered over time about segments of the target audience can be useful in focusing marketing efforts for specific educational activities.

Management of the Marketing Process

- Marketing occurs throughout the educational planning process according to an established timeline.
- The nursing professional development educator assures that all standards and criteria are met in marketing process (e.g., use of accreditation logo and language, commercial support guidelines).
- Implement marketing strategies at established points during the planning process (e.g., save-the-date notice, mailings, announcements, reminders).
- Advertising and publicity
  - Methods of internal promotion
    - Colorful flyers or banner announcements
    - Bulletin board displays
    - Newsletter or electronic news forums
    - E-mail notices and reminders
    - Word of mouth
  - Methods of external promotion
    - Direct mail—brochures, calendars, or catalogs
    - Advertisements—free or paid
    - Word of mouth
    - Web sites
    - E-mail
  - Design of promotional material
    - Design and information may vary for internal and external audiences.
    - Information to be included: title, date, time, location, program purpose, objectives, benefits to participants, target audience, schedule, faculty information, registration information, contact hours, cost, hotel information (if necessary), travel and driving directions (if necessary), parking, disability or dietary accommodations, cancellation and refund policies, and contact information.
    - Design elements to consider: easy-to-read font size and typeface; dark, contrasting color on light background; adequate white space; appealing, personalized format.
    - Promotional materials should be proofread for accuracy, completeness, and clarity of content (Alspach, 1995; Rodriguez, 1996).
  - Use of mailing lists
    - Mailing lists, when used, should be current, accurate, and complete.
    - Mailing lists may be developed using past participant information.
    - Mailing lists may be purchased for target audience from external sources (e.g., ANA, specialty organizations, board of nursing).
- Evaluation of marketing plan
  - Collect data related to elements of marketing plan (e.g., demographic data of participants, how participants heard about or decided to attend activity)
  - Analyze marketing data to determine effectiveness of strategies (e.g., track timing of registrations with mailings, announcements; monitor Web site visits)

- Analyze financial data to determine effectiveness of promotional costs (e.g., percent of revenue spent on promotion; most effective strategies in producing revenue; Alspach, 1995).

MANAGEMENT OF EDUCATIONAL ACTIVITIES

Budgeting

- "The nursing professional development educator develops a financial plan sufficient to meet educational needs" (ANA, 2000, p. 21).
- Definitions
  - *Operational budget* reflects the day-to-day costs of operating a staff development department, including salaries and supplies.
  - *Capital budget* provides for the acquisition of major equipment used over a period of time such as manikins, video equipment, and classroom furniture (Sheridan & Frost-Hartzler, 1996).
  - *Revenue* is income.
  - *Expenditures* are expenses.
  - *Direct costs* are out-of-pocket expenses spent on educational activities (e.g., speaker honorarium, travel, marketing, materials).
  - *Indirect costs* are in-house contributions such as employee salaries and benefits, space, and overhead (e.g., heat, lighting, electricity) costs.
  - *Fixed costs* are costs that remain the same regardless of the amount of business activity (e.g., classroom furniture, speaker honorarium, audiovisual support, initial publicity).
  - *Variable costs* are costs that vary proportionally with the amount of business activity (e.g., printing, refreshments).
  - *Commercial support* is defined as "financial or in-kind contributions given by a commercial interest, which is used to pay all or part of the costs of a CNE activity" (ANCC, 2009).
- Cost–benefit analysis is a process that identifies the economic efficiency of a program in terms of the relationship between costs and benefits (in monetary terms).
  - Itemize costs of the educational activity.
  - Itemize benefits of the educational activity to the learner, the organization, and the patient.
  - Translate costs and benefits into monetary terms.
- Cost-effectiveness analysis is a process that measures the efficiency of achieving outcomes in relation to costs (cost/unit of outcomes achieved).
  - Define realistic, measurable objectives.
  - Determine program costs.
  - Measure learner outcomes to evaluate success (Sheridan & Frost-Hartzler, 1996).
- A budget worksheet is a helpful tool in determining the expenses and revenue associated with an educational activity.
- A completed budget worksheet can be used to determine registration fees for the current and future educational activities.
- ANCC (2009) has adapted a set of *Standards for Disclosure and Commercial Support* that articulates policies for disclosure and commercial support in the planning and provision of continuing nursing education activities.

Policies

- The nursing professional development educator collaborates with others to develop and implement policies that address all relevant aspects of the educational activity. Areas addressed in policy and procedure statements may include:
  - Registration process
  - Cancellation process and fees (if any)
  - Silencing cell phones/pagers
  - Criteria for successful completion
  - Audio- or videotaping
- Learners must be informed in advance of policies that may influence their decision to participate in an educational activity (Aucoin, 1998a).

Process Management

- Preregistration may or may not be required.
- If used, a preregistration process must be developed and clearly communicated to potential participants.
- Preregistration or registration may be managed using a written or electronic form.
- If a fee is involved, communicate the amount and what it covers (e.g., lunch, handouts) to potential participants.
- Have a method to collect fees via cash, check, or credit card.
- Communicate the policy for cancellation of the event to potential participants.
- Include registrant cancellation policies and process, including any deadlines or penalties, in program marketing materials.
- Have a user-friendly registration process available onsite the day of the educational activity (Aucoin, 1998a).

Facility Management

- Select a physical environment that is comfortable for learners, appropriate for the teaching strategies being used, and supportive of the presenter's requirements (Schoenly, 1998).
- Factors to consider in selecting a location for an educational activity:
  - Target audience: Is the activity for an internal audience or targeted to a local, regional, or national audience?
  - Topic, objectives, and teaching strategies: Does the educational activity require skills practice, group work, or tables for note-taking or projects?
  - Availability of audiovisual, computers, and LCD projectors, including cost and availability of technical support
  - Comfortable seating arrangements and room space for the size of the group
  - Adequate lighting and ventilation
  - Ability to control room temperature
  - Minimal background noise or distractions in adjacent areas
  - Availability of restrooms and other needed conveniences
  - Availability of catering services for breaks and meals, if needed
  - Requirements met for Americans With Disabilities Act (ADA)

- Availability of space as needed to accommodate posters, displays, concurrent sessions, breaks, and meals
- Adequate, well-lit, and safe parking areas (Aucoin, 1998b; Aucoin, 2002; Wilkinson, 2002)
- Additional considerations for an external conference being marketed regionally or nationally include:
  - Availability and cost of overnight accommodations
  - Transportation convenience and options
  - Availability of other area attractions
- Once the location has been determined, arrangements and details for room set-up and clean-up must be determined (Aucoin, 1998a).

On-Site Coordination

- Have an adequate number of handouts and other class documents (e.g., registration forms, evaluation forms, certificates of attendance) available onsite.
- Check availability and operation of audiovisual, computer, and other equipment prior to the start of the activity.
- Ensure that refreshments are delivered on time.
- Control environmental factors such as lighting and room temperature.
- If coordinating a large conference or group, arrange to have staff and volunteers available to assist with identified responsibilities (e.g., room monitor, speaker support) to ensure smooth coordination throughout the educational activity.
- Address participant concerns or questions with courtesy and respect.
- Collect evaluation data and distribute certificates of attendance.

Troubleshooting

- Be prepared with a backup plan in case problems arise related to any of the following situations:
  - Speaker illness or unexpected conflict
  - Audiovisual, computer, or other equipment malfunction
  - Unanticipated distractions or interruptions (e.g., construction noise in a hotel, patient care activities near a unit classroom)

REFERENCES

Alspach, J. G. (1995). *The educational process in nursing staff development.* St. Louis, MO: Mosby.

American Nurses Association. (2000). *Scope and standards of practice for nursing professional development.* Washington, DC: American Nurses Publishing.

American Nurses Credentialing Center. (2009). *Application manual: Accreditation program.* Silver Spring, MD: Author.

Aucoin, J. W. (1998a). *101 tips to better conferences.* Pensacola, FL: National Nursing Staff Development Organization.

Aucoin, J. W. (1998b). Program planning: Solving the problem. In K. J. Kelly-Thomas, *Clinical and nursing staff development: Current competence, future focus* (2nd ed., pp. 213–239). Philadelphia: Lippincott.

Aucoin, J. W. (2002). Planning. In B. E. Puetz & J. W. Aucoin (Eds.), *Conversations in nursing professional development* (pp. 151–155). Pensacola, FL: Pohl Publishing.

Rodriguez, L. (1996). In-house marketing of staff development programs. In R. S. Abruzzese (Ed.), *Nursing staff development: Strategies for success* (2nd ed., pp. 142–155). St. Louis, MO: Mosby.

Schoenly, L. (1998). Creating an environment of learning: An opportunity. In K. J. Kelly-Thomas, *Clinical and nursing staff development: Current competence, future focus* (2nd ed., pp. 282–300). Philadelphia: Lippincott.

Sheridan, D. R., & Frost-Hartzler, P. (1996). Documenting effectiveness: Budget and cost considerations. In R. S. Abruzzese (Ed.), *Nursing staff development: Strategies for success* (2nd ed., pp. 122–141). St. Louis, MO: Mosby.

Wilkinson, C. S. (2002). Implementing. In B. E. Puetz & J. W. Aucoin (Eds.), *Conversations in nursing professional development* (pp. 157–170). Pensacola, FL: Pohl Publishing.

Evaluation

BACKGROUND

- Evaluation is a systematic, ongoing process, and is based on specific criteria.
- Educators, learners, content experts, management, and administration are involved in the evaluation process as appropriate.
- Evaluation data are used to revise learning activities to increase their effectiveness.
- The effectiveness of learning activities is directly related to the achievement of learning objectives and impact on job performance.
- Methods and levels of evaluation vary from the learner's response to an educational activity through overall program effectiveness. The level selected supports the organization's culture of learning.
- The method and level of an evaluation is based on the situation: problem, stakeholders, outcome, data sources, tools available, cost, time, and practicality.
- The evaluation data are summarized, documented, and shared, along with outcome achievement, with appropriate individuals, including educators, faculty, content experts, staff members, planning committees, and stakeholders (American Nurses Association [ANA], 2000).

PURPOSES OF EVALUATION

- Evaluation is an organized, thorough assessment of educational endeavors. The purpose of evaluation is to determine the effectiveness of such endeavors and assign value or worth to them.
- It is essential that evaluation be conducted systematically and involve analysis of all activities associated with educational programming.
- The effectiveness of learning activities is evaluated in relation to the "development of the individual nurse's portfolio, which includes documentation of ongoing professional development, career planning, and continuing professional development" (ANA, 2000, p. 15).
- A goal of evaluation is to improve the effectiveness of educational programming.
- The results of evaluation are used to identify future educational needs, appropriate faculty, and effective teaching and learning methodologies.
- Evaluation also is conducted for meeting the standards of accrediting organizations.
- Evaluation is imperative for the calculation of the cost–benefit ratio of specific learning activities (Avillion, 2005; Kirkpatrick, 1998).

Types of Evaluation

- *Competency-based evaluation:* Assessment of a nurse's demonstrated ability to satisfactorily achieve specific behaviors essential to the role of the nurse and requirements of the job description. For example, assessment against all competency statements and performance criteria for a specific role during an orientation period.
- *Criterion-referenced evaluation:* Evaluation of behaviors against a set of specific, predetermined criteria. For example, attained passing score or not; American Heart Association's Basic Cardiac Life Support course performance checklists for single rescuer. obstructed airway, and so on.
- *Norm-referenced evaluation:* Evaluation of the achievement of a learner compared to that of other learners, reported as scores or percentages. For example, grading on a curve, the Scholastic Aptitude Test (SAT).
- *Formative evaluation:* Evaluation that takes place during the learning activity and is used to alter content or methods of teaching. For example, periodic meetings with preceptors and orientees to determine progress, learner self-assessments on their progress.
- *Summative evaluation:* Evaluation that occurs upon completion of the learning activity and is used to determine learner outcomes and activity effectiveness. For example, certification, budget reports of cost-effectiveness.
- *Program evaluation:* Consideration of various components of an overall educational plan and process (Alspach, 1995).

METHODOLOGIES OF EVALUATION

Kirkpatrick's Four Levels (Kirkpatrick, 1998)

- *Level 1: Reaction.* The measure of customer satisfaction; sometimes referred to as a "happiness" index. Reaction is essentially the learner's response to the effectiveness of the educator, teaching or learning method, and learning environment, and how well the program was perceived to meet the learning objectives.
- *Level 2: Learning.* The extent to which learners acquire knowledge and skills or change attitudes. Learning requires measurement of objective achievement.
- *Level 3: Behavior.* The extent to which behavioral changes occur after participating in a learning activity. In addition to presenting an effective education program, other conditions must be met for behavior to change. The learner must want to change, know how and what to do, work in a setting that facilitates the change, and be rewarded for implementing the change.
- *Level 4: Results.* The effect the learning activity has on the measures that are important to the organization. Examples of desired results include a decrease in the number of medication errors, decreased staff attrition, an increase in patient satisfaction, or a decrease in the number of nosocomial infections.
- Because many other factors can impact organizational effectiveness, the time and resources devoted to evaluation should relate to the benefits of the evaluation.
- Kirkpatrick's model serves as the basis for many evaluation systems.

RSA Model

- Developed by Roberta S. Abruzzese for the purpose of conceptualizing evaluations, the RSA model consists of five levels of education and measurement:
  - *Level 1: Process.* Measures the learner's general satisfaction with the faculty, program content, how well the content met stated objectives, teaching and learning methodologies, and the learning environment.
  - *Level 2: Content.* Assesses changes in the learner's knowledge, skill, or attitudes after completing a learning activity.
  - *Level 3: Outcome.* Evaluates changes in the learner's actual nursing practice in the work setting after the completion of a learning activity.
  - *Level 4: Impact.* Measures organization outcomes that can be attributed, in part, to the effects of a learning experience.
  - *Level 5: Total Program.* Evaluates the congruence of goals, objectives, accomplishments, and outcomes (Abruzzese, 1996).

CIPP Model

- Developed by D. L. Stufflebeam (2003), the CIPP (Context, Input, Process, Product) model examines four aspects of projects and programs for both formative and summative evaluation.
- Most notably used for program and system process evaluations.

- **Context:** Assesses data that deal with planning and determining goals, objectives, and priorities. *Formative:* What needs to be done? *Summative:* Were important needs addressed?
- **Input:** Evaluates internal and external resources, approaches, plans, and goals in relation to feasibility and effectiveness. Data from input evaluation is used for decision-making. *Formative:* How should it be done? *Summative:* Was the effort guided by a defensible plan and budget?
- **Process:** Assesses implementation of plan (decided from *Input* evaluation) to judge performance and outcomes. *Formative:* Is it being done? *Summative:* Was the service design executed competently and modified as needed?
- **Product:** Identifies and assesses outcomes in meeting targeted needs. *Formative:* Is it succeeding? *Summative:* Did the effort succeed?

Three-Step Evaluation Model

- Designed by Wagner and Weigand (2002) as a more pragmatic method of training evaluation.
  - *Step 1.* Determine the staff behavior that is to result from the training. This should be done collaboratively between the manager and the training department.
  - *Step 2.* Identify the possible organizational improvements as a result of the staff behavior changes. This can be done by a small group of managers and/or trainers.
  - *Step 3.* Link the behavior change to results that are already being measured in the organization. This is best done by management with the assistance of financial experts who have access to data that others may not know exists.
  - "The newly discovered data might be the missing link that is needed for measuring training results" (Wagner & Weigand, 2002, p. 121).

Accreditation Evaluation Model

- This model is used for program evaluation.
- Accrediting bodies such as The Joint Commission and American Nurses Credentialing Center (ANCC) develop standards and criteria.
- Effectiveness of education programs is evaluated according to these standards and criteria.
- Accreditation depends, in part, on how well education programs meet these standards and criteria.
- Accreditation involves four steps:
  1. The program mission, goals, and desired outcomes are established.
  2. A self-paced study exercise is conducted to assess how well standards and criteria are being met.
  3. A review process that includes document reviews and stakeholder interviews is conducted by an external peer group.
  4. The independent accrediting body representatives read the self-paced study and peer review documents and make accreditation recommendations (ANCC, 2006; Dickerson, 2002).

TOOLS OF EVALUATION

- Various tools and resources are required to collect necessary evaluation data.
- Examples of tools and resources are:
  - Self-rating scales
  - Pre- and posttests
  - Return demonstration in a simulated setting
  - Competency assessment forms
  - Direct observation in the clinical setting
  - Medical record review
  - Review of quality improvement data
  - Review of risk management data
  - Review of patient, staff, and/or physician satisfaction surveys
  - Data from performance evaluations
  - Results of accreditation and/or regulatory surveys (Avillion, 2005; Kelly-Thomas, 1998).

USE OF EVALUATION DATA

The Kirkpatrick (1998) and Abruzzese (1996) models will be used to discuss the use of evaluation data.

Evaluating Reaction/Process Data

- It is important to obtain learner reaction regardless of the method of teaching and learning.
- The level of learner satisfaction can be correlated to the learner's level of motivation and interest in learning (Kirkpatrick, 1998).
- Reaction evaluation data are just as important as other levels of evaluation and should not be discounted; reaction evaluations help to identify effective teaching styles and methods (Avillion, 2005, 2008; Kirkpatrick, 1998).
- Data from reaction/process evaluations are reviewed for trends with revisions to the content, delivery method, or curriculum made accordingly.

Evaluating Learning/Content

- Positive reactions to a particular learning event are important, but do not indicate actual knowledge acquisition.
- Learning is measured by comparing knowledge, skills, or attitudes prior to and after completing an education program.
- Start by constructing well-written objectives that measure learning, such as "After completing this self-learning module, the learner accurately calculates pediatric medication doses based on a patient's weight in kilograms 100% of the time."
- The type of evaluation is based on the learning domains of the objectives. (See Chapter 3.)

- A paper and pencil test is the most common form of learning/content evaluation for the cognitive domain. The test also may be delivered via computer.
- Pretests administered immediately prior to the program give both educators and learners the opportunity to assess current knowledge, and pretests can increase learner motivation.
- Note that if a nurse completes a well-written pretest (see Test Construction, Chapter 11) successfully, she or he may not need to complete the learning activity.
- This tactic is especially useful during orientation; pretests can be developed to serve as "challenge" exams.
- Successful completion of such exams may allow orientees to avoid sitting in the classroom or participating in distance learning programs and move through orientation more quickly.
- These types of exams also may be built into competency programs.
- This strategy helps to acknowledge levels of expertise and helps nurses to pursue the education they need, rather than education that is unnecessary or redundant.
- Examples of other ways of measuring knowledge acquisition include the use of case studies, group activities, simulations, and demonstration.
- The formality of learning/content evaluation is based on the purpose of the learning activity (Avillion, 2005, 2008; Kirkpatrick, 1998).

Evaluating Behavior/Outcome

- It is not enough to demonstrate learning as a result of an educational activity.
- If learners fail to apply what they have learned, the effectiveness of education is compromised.
- Evaluating behavior involves the compilation of data to measure behavioral changes in the clinical setting as a result of participation in a learning activity.
- Some may think that as long as learning occurs, and employees are motivated to apply what they have learned in the work setting, desired behavior will take place. However, a number of barriers may prevent implementation of desired behaviors. These barriers must be addressed prior to attempting to initiate behavioral changes.
  - Management resistance to behavioral change: Managers must recognize why the behavioral changes are necessary and important, and support the implementation of such changes. Managers who fail to recognize and support the application of new knowledge as evidenced by behavioral changes may covertly or overtly hinder staff members' ability to initiate change.
  - Lack of necessary resources: If necessary resources (e.g., computers, patient care equipment) are not available to implement new behaviors, not only will staff be unable to apply knowledge, they will doubt the value and worth of future learning activities.
  - Employee resistance: Employees who do not recognize the value and worth of behavioral change or who fear change may overtly or covertly sabotage implementation of behavioral change.
  - Multiple overlapping priorities: The numerous behavior changes required do not allow the learner time to incorporate the behavior change as part of daily practice.
- Those who evaluate behavioral change (e.g., peers, managers, educators) must do so consistently.
- Evaluators should follow a written set of guidelines that explicitly identify what constitutes appropriate behavioral change.
- Results of these evaluations should be shared with the person evaluated, strengths acknowledged, and, if necessary, an action plan for improvement initiated.

- The form used to document this type of evaluation should have a place for the signatures of the evaluator and the person evaluated, as well as the results of the evaluation.
- If the person being evaluated fails to perform the desired behavior appropriately, the action plan (including objectives and desired date of achievement) should be documented on the evaluation form and signed by both the evaluator and the person being evaluated.
- This type of documentation provides a written record of the steps necessary to achieve the objectives.
- Ways to evaluate behavior include direct observation, peer review, medical record review, and patient outcomes (Avillion, 2008; Ludeman, 1998).

Evaluating Results/Impact

- Evaluation of impact is the process of assessing the results of education that affect organizational functioning.
- The data collected when evaluating behavioral change or application of learning form the basis for impact evaluation:
  - For example, suppose risk management and quality improvement data show a significant increase in the occurrence of nosocomial infections. The causes of these infections have been traced to lack of hand washing, failure to maintain sterile techniques, and failure to initiate antibiotic therapy when the patients' conditions indicated the existence of an infection.
  - Extensive education offerings were presented to all direct patient care providers.
  - In addition to evaluating reaction, knowledge acquisition was measured by pre- and posttests and case studies.
  - Behavioral change was assessed by direct observation, medical record audits, and review of patient care plans.
  - Impact was measured by statistical comparison of the type, number, and cause of nosocomial infections three months before and three months after the educational offerings.
  - Improvement was calculated in percentages and evaluated in terms of the total organization, by department, and by unit.
- The results of this level of evaluation should be shared with staff, management, and appropriate stakeholders (e.g., infection control, quality improvement, risk management; Avillion, 2005; Shelton & Alliger, 1998).

Return on Investment (ROI)

- The purpose of evaluating ROI is to measure the effect of education on the financial bottom line.
- The assumption with ROI is that benefit can be quantified and training is the sole variable in achieving that benefit.
- This type of evaluation is complex and takes considerable time and effort.
- ROI is not calculated on every learning activity, but only on those that have the most significant impact on organizational effectiveness.
- Two measures are used for this high level of education evaluation: cost/benefit ratio and return on investment formula.

- Both measures use annual values because the value of short-term training is most frequently captured within a year (Phillips, 1997).
- Cost/benefit ratio (CBR) compares the economic benefit (expressed in dollars) of a program to the cost of the program. The organization establishes an acceptable cost/benefit ratio standard. The formula is:

$$CBR = \frac{Program\ Benefits}{Program\ Costs}$$

- Return on investment (ROI) is the benefits (expressed in dollars) minus the costs of a learning activity. The difference is divided by the costs, then multiplied by 100 so that the ROI is expressed as a percentage:

$$ROI\ (\%) = \frac{(Benefits - Costs)}{Costs} \times 100$$

- Consider the example in the preceding section concerning the need to decrease the incidence of nosocomial infections. It would be necessary to determine the expenses directly related to the increased rate of nosocomial infections.
  - Expenses include increased length of stay, loss of third-party reimbursement, cost of additional diagnostic procedures and treatments triggered by nosocomial infections, and the cost of any damages paid to the patient or family as a result of malpractice lawsuits related to such infections. Also included are the costs of developing, implementing, and evaluating the learning activities designed to decrease the incidence of nosocomial infections.
  - The benefits include the money saved as a result of decreased length of stay when no nosocomial infections develop, no expenses for additional diagnostic and treatment measures, appropriate third-party reimbursement, and lack of malpractice awards.
- ROI demonstrates the financial worth of a learning activity in terms of business and strategic goals. Educational programs specifically done to impact an organization's profits are most suited for an ROI evaluation (Avillion, 2005; Kirkpatrick, 1998; Phillips, 1997).

OUTCOME MEASURES

Cost/benefit ratio, ROI, and results/impact evaluation are types of outcome measures. However, in health care other performance measures are considered outcomes measures.

Benchmarking

- Benchmarking is the comparison of an organization with one or more organizations or data sets that are considered experts or leaders.
- Benchmarking can be performed with a primary competitor, internally among different departments, with organizations of similar size and scope, or with award-winning organizations.

- It is an effective means to identify improvements that can make a significant difference to an organization.
- Benchmarking is done to improve the efficiency or effectiveness of a process to produce the desired outcome. The focus is the process, not the result.
- The benchmark is the "ideal" and can be used for a gap analysis, with the educational program designed to bridge that gap.
- Program outcome effectiveness is indirectly related to changes against the benchmark.
- Examples of benchmark data that can be impacted by educational programs are staff vacancy rate, infection rates, employee satisfaction, and quality indicators (Kelly-Thomas, 1998; Marrelli, 1997).

Quality Indicators

- Quality Indicators (QIs) provide a perspective on the quality of care provided by hospitals.
- The Agency for Healthcare Research and Quality (AHRQ) and the Centers for Medicare & Medicaid Services (CMS) set the initial QIs and continues to add to them.
- QIs are publicly reported by hospitals.
- QIs can assist hospitals to identify problem areas for further review of processes that affect the outcome measure.
- Examples of QIs are mortality rates for stroke and hip replacements, number of hysterectomies, pneumococcal and influenza vaccination status of patients with pneumonia, perioperative urinary catheter removal by postoperative day 2, and re-admissions for heart failure (AHRQ, 2006; CMS, 2010).

Performance Measures

- The organization selects which measures will become part of its continual performance monitoring.
- Tools used for performance monitoring and quality improvement processes include dashboards, scorecards, and report cards.
- The purpose of these tools is to keep the performance measures in the forefront of everyday practice.
- The sophistication of the tool depends on the resources of the organization. Data can be displayed in traditional charts, graphs, or other indicators such as color-coded grids or gauges.
- When process improvements are identified, education/training is most frequently the mechanism employed for correction. However, most process improvements are not corrected by an educational activity. Rather, the educational activity teaches the employee what behavior changes are needed to improve the organization's desired outcome.
- Examples of performance measures are quality indicators, national patient safety goals, and core measures.

REFERENCES

Abruzzese, R. S. (Ed.). (1996). *Nursing staff development: Strategies for success.* St. Louis, MO: Mosby.

Agency for Healthcare Research and Quality. (2006). *Inpatient quality indicators overview.* Rockville, MD: Author. Retrieved from http://www.qualityindicators.ahrq.gov/iqi_overview.htm

American Nurses Association. (2000). *Scope and standards of practice for nursing professional development.* Washington, DC: American Nurses Publishing.

American Nurses Credentialing Center. (2006). *Manual for accreditation as an approver or provider of continuing nursing education: Application manual.* Silver Spring, MD: American Nurses Credentialing Center.

Avillion, A. E. (2005). *Nurse educator manual: Essential skills and guidelines for effective practice.* Marblehead, MA: HCPro.

Avillion, A. E. (2008). *A practical guide to staff development: Tools and techniques for effective education* (2nd ed.). Marblehead, MA: HCPro.

Centers for Medicaid & Medicare Services. (2010). *Reporting hospital quality data for annual payment update.* Retrieved from https://www.cms.gov/HospitalQualityInits/08_HospitalRHQDAPU.asp

Dickerson, P. S. (2002). Accreditation/approval criteria. In B. E. Puetz & J. W. Aucoin (Eds.), *Conversations in nursing professional development* (pp. 187–193). Pensacola, FL: Pohl Publishing.

Kelly-Thomas, K. J. (1998). *Clinical and nursing staff development: Current competence, future focus* (2nd ed.). Philadelphia: Lippincott.

Kirkpatrick, D. L. (1998). *Evaluating training programs* (2nd ed.). San Francisco: Berrett-Koehler.

Ludeman, K. (1998). Measuring skills and behavior. In D. L. Kirkpatrick, *Another look at evaluating training programs* (pp. 154–158). Alexandria, VA: American Society for Training & Development.

Marelli, T. M. (1997). *The nurse manager's survival guide: Practical answers to everyday problems* (2nd ed.). St. Louis, MO: Mosby.

Phillips, J. J. (1997). *Handbook of training evaluation and measurement methods* (3rd ed.). Oxford, UK: Elsevier.

Shelton, S., & Alliger, G. (1998). Who's afraid of level 4 evaluation? A practical approach. In D. L. Kirkpatrick, *Another look at evaluating training programs* (pp. 171–174). Alexandria, VA: American Society for Training & Development.

Stufflebeam, D. L. (2003). *The CIPP model for evaluation.* Retrieved from http://www.oregoneval.org/program/CIPP%20Model%20for%20Evaluation.pdf

Wagner, R. J., & Weigand, R. (2002). Measuring the organizational impact of training programs. In P. L. Spath (Ed.), *Guide to effective staff development in health care organizations: A systems approach to successful training* (pp. 113–125). San Francisco: Jossey-Bass.

12

Documentation and Records

BACKGROUND

- Each Standard of Practice for Nursing Professional Development (American Nurses Association [ANA], 2000) refers to documentation:
  - Assessment: "Relevant data are documented in a retrievable form" (p. 12)
  - Diagnosis: "Identified needs are documented in a manner that facilitates the determination of purpose statements, educational objectives, program content, and evaluation data" (p. 13)
  - Planning: "The outline of the content is documented" (p. 14)
  - Implementation: "Criteria for successful completion of the educational activity are provided to the learner and are documented" (p. 14)
  - Evaluation: "A summary of the evaluation responses and achievement of outcomes is documented and shared with the appropriate persons, such as content experts, presenters, and the planning committee" (p. 15)
- Standard VIII, Management and Resource Utilization, under Standards of Professional Performance for Nursing Professional Development (ANA, 2000), has the measurement criteria:
  - "Maintains a record-keeping and report system that
    - Documents all aspects of educational activities in compliance with departmental, organizational, and external agency requirements.

- Establishes mechanisms for systematic, easy retrieval of data on educational activities and participants.
- Maintains confidentiality of records.
- Provides periodic reports to appropriate organizational and agency representatives to document and evaluate progress toward attainment of organizational goals." (p. 21)

RECORD MANAGEMENT

Purposes

- Monitor instructional programs for their relevance, effectiveness, and efficiency.
- Comply with established educational standards, accreditation standards, state laws, and licensing regulations.
- Convey information about nursing professional development program to relevant groups who use information for planning, managing, and decision-making.
  - External audiences: National accrediting and regulatory agencies, such as The Joint Commission, American Nurses Credentialing Center (ANCC), Occupational Safety and Health Administration (OSHA), state boards of nursing, and state departments of health
  - Internal audiences: Administrator of organization, nursing director, nursing professional development unit personnel (Alspach, 1995)

Types of Records

- Job requirement: Requisites for employment such as license, certificates (e.g., BLS, FHM, ACLS, NRP), occupational health (e.g., vaccinations, titers, TB screening)
- Orientation: Documents for new employee as well as change in roles, responsibilities, and/ or practice settings within an organization that indicate how competency was assessed and requirement was met
- Ongoing competency: Record of attendance at mandatory training and validation of competency to mitigate risk
- Continuing education: Attendance and completion of internal or external educational activities that further knowledge and skills in profession, role, and/or practice area

Maintenance of Records

- Educational records can be kept manually or via computer software applications.
- Have a back-up (hard copy and/or electronic) so documents are retrievable should there be a natural or unnatural disaster.
- Organizations may set policies and guidelines for maintaining records, including how long records need to be kept.
- Responsibility for educational records may be with the employee, management, or both.
- Educational records may be embedded in a learning management system.
- Records may be arranged chronologically, alphabetically, or by topic area. Consistency is key in being able to retrieve documents for review and reporting.

- Retrieval of documents may be for performance review, accreditation, risk management, and compliance reports for regulatory agencies.
- Access to records is on a need-to-know basis. Confidentiality is guided by organizational human resource and education department policies.
- Sophisticated automated systems may include bar-code scanning for employee identification badges, link to time and attendance records, or performance evaluation systems (Kelly-Thomas, 1998; O'Shea, 2002).

ACCREDITATION DOCUMENTATION

- Foundational documents for the ANCC accreditation system (ANCC, 2009):
  - *Scope and Standards of Practice for Nursing Professional Development* (ANA, 2000)
  - *Code of Ethics for Nurses with Interpretive Statements* (ANA, 2001)
  - Adult learning principles and behavioral objectives from teaching–learning principles, educational theory, and pedagogical literature (ANCC, 2009).
- A provider unit has one or more designated nurse planners responsible for being involved with the entire process of an educational activity and documenting adherence to ANCC Accreditation Program criteria (ANCC, 2009).
- Documentation of the following is required for nursing continuing education activities:
  - Title, location, and date of educational activity
  - Assessment of learner needs
  - Target audience
  - Qualifications of planning committee planners and presenters
  - Conflict of interest disclosure statements
  - Effective design principles
  - Process used to verify participation
  - Notice to learners how successful completion will be measured
  - Marketing and promotional material
  - Coprovider and commercial support agreements
  - Evaluation tools including a summary evaluation
  - Contact hour credits
  - Sample certificate of completion
  - Participant names and addresses (ANCC, 2009)
- Education design components include:
  - An identified purpose of the educational activity
  - Explicit, measurable educational objectives for the learner
  - Content congruent with the activity's purpose and educational objectives
  - Teaching and learning strategies congruent to the activity's objectives and content
  - Evaluation strategy consistent with objectives and content
  - Criteria for judging successful completion of an activity (Alspach, 1995; ANCC, 2009; Dickerson, 2002)
- ANCC (2009) requires records be kept in a secure and confidential manner for a period of 6 years.

REFERENCES

Alspach, J. G. (1995). *The educational process in nursing staff development.* St. Louis, MO: Mosby.

American Nurses Association. (2000). *Scope and standards of practice for nursing professional development.* Washington, DC: American Nurses Publishing.

American Nurses Association. (2001). *Code of ethics for nurses with interpretive statements.* Washington, DC: American Nurses Publishing.

American Nurses Credentialing Center. (2009). *Application manual: Accreditation program.* Silver Spring, MD: Author.

Dickerson, P. (2002). *Accreditation/approval criteria.* In B. E. Puetz & J. W. Aucoin (Eds.), *Conversations in nursing professional development* (pp. 187–193). Pensacola, FL: Pohl Publishing.

Kelly-Thomas, K. J. (1998). *Clinical and nursing staff development: Current competence, future focus* (2nd ed.). Philadelphia: Lippincott.

O'Shea, K. L. (2002). *Staff development nursing secrets.* Philadelphia: Hanley & Belfus.

13

Communication

BACKGROUND

- In the *Scope and Standards of Practice for Nursing Professional Development* (American Nurses Association [ANA], 2000), Standard IV, Collegiality, requires the nursing professional development educator to interact with peers and other healthcare providers, share knowledge and skills, and provide constructive feedback to peers regarding their practice. These activities require communication skills.
- "Communicating efficiently and effectively with all levels of the organization and using problem solving skills are other aspects of the leadership role" (ANA, 2000, p. 10).

Listening Skills

- Realize that listening is an active process that requires skill, discipline, and practice.
- Concentrate on the words and behavior of the speaker without passing judgment.
- Be supportive of self-expression.
- Be aware that the goal of listening is to understand.
- Listen with genuine interest.
- Minimize distractions.

- Establish and maintain eye contact, giving full attention to the speaker.
- Paraphrase as needed to clarify.
- NEVER interrupt.
- Pay attention to nonverbal communication (Harvey & Sims, 2003).

Communication Tips

- Watch language; avoid technical terms and acronyms that might not be understood by all.
- Use fewer words.
- Avoid "data dumps"—keep communications to no more than three key points.
- Use visual messages.
- Get feedback from staff members.
- Use communication to build "USA": understanding, support, and acceptance.
- Communicate purpose and listen without prejudice (Harvey & Sims, 2003; LaBarre, 2004).

Potential Barriers to Effective Organizational Communication

- Time pressures
- Environmental interference
- Lack of information
- Faulty reasoning
- Organizational complexity
- Selective perception
- Research has shown that 75% of all management problems result from poor communication (Grant & Massey, 1999).

NEGOTIATION SKILLS

- Definitions
  - Networking: "Aligning oneself with others to obtain information, ideas, advice, power, and influence" (Zimmerman & Jones, 2002, p. 167)
  - Consensus-building: Pre–decision-making process of informal meetings, discussion, and agreements on issues on a personal level; an effective form of negotiation
  - Negotiation: Dialogue process in which two or more parties compromise to reach agreement on course of action to meet synergistic goals and objectives
- Negotiation requires input and compromise from stakeholders.
- The most effective negotiation process has a win-win outcome (Zimmerman & Jones, 2002).

Principled Negotiation

- Principled negotiation decides issues on their merits, looks for mutual gains, and insists on fair standards. There are four basic points to principled negotiations:
  1. Separate the people from the problem; understand others' thinking.
  2. Focus on interests instead of positions; look for shared and compatible interests as well as conflicting ones.
  3. Generate a variety of options before deciding what to do; brainstorm first without judging ideas, then evaluate and decide on the best options.
  4. Insist that the result be based on an objective standard (Fisher & Ury, 1991).

Negotiating Strategies With Various Individuals

Adversaries—low agreement and low trust
Opponents—low agreement and high trust
Allies—high agreement and high trust
Bedfellows—high agreement and low trust

- Strategies for dealing with adversaries
  - State the vision of the project.
  - State in a neutral way your own best understanding of the adversary's position.
  - Identify your own contributions to the problem.
  - End the meeting with your own plans and no demand.
- Strategies for dealing with opponents
  - Reaffirm the quality of the relationship and mutual trust.
  - State your own position.
  - State in a neutral way what you believe to be the opponent's position.
  - Problem-solve.
- Strategies for dealing with allies
  - Affirm agreement.
  - Reaffirm the quality of the trusting relationship.
  - Acknowledge doubts and vulnerabilities related to the project.
  - Ask for advice and support.
- Strategies for dealing with bedfellows
  - Reaffirm the agreement.
  - Acknowledge caution.
  - Be clear about what one wants from the bedfellow.
  - Ask what the bedfellow wants and expects.
  - Try to agree about how to work together (Marriner-Tomey, 2004).

TEAM-BUILDING

- "Team building is an intentional process" (Chitty & Black, 2010, p. 219).
- The nursing professional development educator models team-building behaviors: shows respect to others, builds trust, identifies problematic feelings and misperceptions and corrects them, involves team members in decision-making, and promotes a caring and supportive practice (Chitty & Black, 2010).

Characteristics of Cultures That Support Teams

- Value employees' need for relationships with others.
- Promote cooperative rather than competitive relationships.
- Encourage individual accountability and responsibility.
- Recognize individual contributions.
- Have positive visions of the future.
- Have short- and long-term goals.
- Have quality standards.
- Believe in their products and services.
- Are people-oriented.
- Support the community (Marriner-Tomey, 2004).

Group Development

- Phases are inevitable and necessary for teams to grow, solve problems, and produce results.
- Teams may revert to earlier stages in response to changing circumstances such as change in leadership.
- *Forming:* The first stage of team-building; the task is one of orientation; members are dependent on the leader.
- *Storming:* Different ideas compete for consideration; emotional response to task demands; members resist group influence.
- *Norming:* Trust begins and motivation increases; open exchange of personal opinions; cohesiveness develops.
- *Performing:* Constructive action; group energy is focused on the task; group interpersonal structure is functional.
- *Adjourning:* Mourning; completion of task with group disengaging; may lead to transformational synergy in performance (Tuckman, 2001).

Skills Needed by Teams

- Honesty (articulate current reality openly; identify what is really happening versus what members wish were happening)
- Ability to organize and run effective meetings by assigning roles, establishing ground rules for conduct, setting procedures to follow, and following a written agenda

- Using team-building activities such as courtesy, improving communication, becoming better able to perform everyday work tasks together, and building strong relationships to develop cohesiveness
- Creating an environment that promotes learning, which leads to a shared understanding and effective problem-solving (Gloe, 1998)

Benefits of Self-Managed Teams

- Increased productivity
- Commitment to the organization and to the job
- Common commitment to goals and values
- Shared ownership and responsibility for tasks
- Proactive approach to problems
- Faster response to change
- Flexible work practices
- Motivation through peer pressure rather than management mandates
- Increased employee satisfaction
- Better work climate (Marriner-Tomey, 2004)

COLLABORATION

Definition

- Collaboration is not just cooperation, but the concerted effort of individuals and groups to achieve a shared goal.
- Collaboration requires mutual trust, recognition, and respect among the healthcare team, shared decision-making about patient care, and open dialogue among all parties who have an interest in and concern for health outcomes (ANA, 2001).

Strategies for Successful Collaboration

- Develop collegial relationships with managers to identify staff learning needs and assure management follow-up.
- Learn to relate to nursing staff in a nonthreatening, supportive manner.
- Develop close rapport with nursing staff.
- Find out what motivates staff members to improve their performance, so leader can awaken their motivation.
- Listen carefully to the messages received from manager, staff members, and colleagues; clarify and validate them (Lewis & Case, 2001).

Interdisciplinary Collaboration

- Step one: Together the parties define and redefine the problem; bring perspective of those not present.
- Step two: Analyze the criteria necessary for each discipline that make for an effective solution.
- Step three: All parties bring their criteria to the table.
- Step four: The group generates solutions according to the criteria, selects the solution to implement, and evaluates the results (Case, 2002).

FEEDBACK

- Definition: "Specific knowledge given to participants of learning results" (Ellis & O'Connell, 2009, p. 60).
- Feedback is a critical requirement of sustained high-level performance.
- A lack of feedback leads to unsatisfactory performance.
- Specific, frequent feedback is the quickest, cheapest, and most effective intervention for improving performance.

Characteristics of Feedback

- Starts with clear expectations.
- Specific, not general. For example, "Your documentation was clear, thorough, and concise" rather than "Your documentation was good."
- Given as close to the event as possible.
- Content addresses correct performance.
- Focus is on behavior, not the person.
- Provided sincerely and honestly with an intent to help.
- Shares information and observations, not advice.
- Feedback discussion begins with a specific statement of the problem with expected performance.
- Focuses on "next time" rather than looking backward.

Types of Feedback

- *Negative* feedback consists of put-downs, is not useful, and is typically nonspecific.
- *Neutral* feedback is a statement of a problem with no direction toward improvement.
- *Positive* feedback is a specific statement of what and how performance was done well.
- *Constructive* feedback provides direction for how to improve performance.
- *Recognition* feedback (i.e., a job well done) is a powerful motivator (Fournies, 2000; Peters, 2000).

POSITIVISM

Appreciative Inquiry

- Look for what works in an organization.
- Construct statements of what could be, based on what has been.
- Collective strengths can transform an organization.
- Memories of positive occurrences create a positive energy within the organization.
- Guiding principles:
  - Words create worlds.
  - Positive images lead to positive action.
  - Quality relationships are essential to organizational success.
  - Previously hidden possibilities emerge when an organization engages in conversations that matter.
- The 4-D cycle enables employees to contribute via service to the organization creating positive potential.
  1. Discovery: Search to understand the best of what is and has been.
  2. Dream: Engage in thinking big, out of the box.
  3. Design: Make choices for transformation.
  4. Destiny: Focus on personal and organizational commitments (Cooperrider & Whitney, 2005).
- Examples of appreciative questions:
  - What do you love the most about being a preceptor? (Discovery)
  - What would make for better patient safety? (Dream)
  - What areas do you think most affect patient care? (Design)
  - How would you personally like to be involved in the unit's self-governance? (Destiny)

Positive Communication Skills

- Be attentive and listen.
- Start communication with positive comments.
- Talk in a common language.
- Respect each other's viewpoints and opinions.
- Use body language to show interest.
- Do not play the blame game.
- Conduct communication at the proper time and place.

CONFLICT MANAGEMENT

General Information on Conflict

- Conflict is as inevitable as change.
- Conflict is not always negative; it can be a powerful impetus for positive change.
- Conflicts result from a disparity between real or perceived goals, values, roles, attitudes, or actions of two or more persons or groups.
- Conflict may be individual (within one person), interpersonal (between two or more persons), intragroup (within a group), or intergroup (between two or more groups).
- Managing conflict is highly individualized, but skills in this area are critical for nurses (Grant & Massey, 1999).

Framework for Conflict Assessment

PEPRS Framework
- **Persons:** Identify all involved parties, including their perceptions of the conflict, gender, socioeconomic background, cultural background, and professional socialization.
- **Events and issues:** Develop a clear picture of the triggering events; the surrounding historical context; the level of interdependence among the participants; the issues, goals, and resources; and previously considered solutions.
- **Power:** Assess the impact of power on the conflict; all conflicts are based on attempts to protect participants' self-esteem or change perceived inequities in power because most participants believe that the other person or persons have the greater power in the situation.
- **Regulation:** Resources potentially available to regulate the conflict, including internal and external factors, previous resolution attempts, or a neutral third party.
- **Style:** Be cognizant of the influence of the conflict management style used (Sportsman, 2005).

Modes of Conflict Management
- The Thomas-Kilmann Conflict Mode Instrument looks at two dimensions of behavior: assertiveness ("extent to which the person attempts to satisfy his own concerns") and cooperativeness ("extent to which the person attempts to satisfy the other person's concerns").
- These two dimensions define five different modes of response to conflict:
1. Competing: Assertive and uncooperative; pursues own concerns at the other person's expense
2. Accommodating: Unassertive and cooperative; neglects own concerns to satisfy others' concerns; complete opposite of competing mode
3. Avoiding: Unassertive and uncooperative; pursues neither one's own or others' concerns
4. Collaborating: Assertive and cooperative; works with others to satisfy their concerns; complete opposite of avoiding
5. Compromising: Moderately assertive and moderately cooperative; finds mutually acceptable solution to both parties' concerns
- We are capable of all five modes, but typically rely on the modes with which we are most adept based on temperament or practice (Thomas & Kilmann, 2007).

REFERENCES

American Nurses Association. (2000). *Scope and standards of practice for nursing professional development.* Washington, DC: American Nurses Publishing.

American Nurses Association. (2001). *Code of ethics for nurses with interpretive statements.* Washington, DC: American Nurses Publishing.

Case, B. (2002). Critical thinking. In B. E. Puetz & J. W. Aucoin (Eds.), *Conversations in nursing professional development* (pp. 239–254). Pensacola, FL: Pohl Publishing.

Chitty, K. K., & Black, B. P. (2010). *Professional nursing: Concepts and challenges* (6th ed.). Maryland Heights, MD: Saunders Elsevier.

Cooperrider, D. L., & Whitney, D. (2005). *Appreciative inquiry: A positive revolution in change.* San Francisco: Berrett-Koehler Publishers.

Ellis, N. F., & O'Connell, K. M. (2009). Principles of adult learning. In S. L. Bruce (Ed.), *Core curriculum for staff development* (3rd ed., pp. 33–65). Pensacola, FL: National Nursing Staff Development Organization.

Fisher, R., & Ury, W. (1991). *Getting to yes: Negotiating agreement without giving in* (2nd ed., B. Patton, Ed.). New York: Penguin Books.

Fournies, F. F. (2000). *Coaching for improved work performance* (rev. ed.). New York: McGraw-Hill.

Gloe, D. (1998). Quality management: A staff development tradition. In K. J. Kelley-Thomas (Ed.), *Clinical and nursing staff development: Current competence, future focus* (2nd ed., pp. 301–336). Philadelphia: Lippincott-Raven.

Grant, A. B., & Massey, V. H. (1999). *Nursing leadership, management, and research.* Springhouse, PA: Springhouse.

Harvey, E., & Sims, P. (2003). *Nuts'n bolts leadership: "How to" strategies and practical tips for leaders at ALL levels.* Dallas, TX: Walk the Talk.

LaBarre, P. (2004). The agenda—grassroots leadership. In G. M. Spreitzer & K. H. Perttula (Eds.), *Wiley/Fast Company reader series: Leadership* (pp. 49–56). Hoboken, NJ: Wiley.

Lewis, D. J., & Case, B. (2001). The staff development specialist role. In A. E. Avillion (Ed.), *Core curriculum for staff development* (2nd ed., pp. 91–105). Pensacola, FL: National Nursing Staff Development Organization.

Marriner-Tomey, A. (2004). *Guide to nursing management and leadership* (7th ed.). St Louis, MO: Mosby-Year Book.

Peters, P. (2000). *Seven tips for delivering performance feedback.* Retrieved from http://www.performance-appraisals.org/cgi-bin/links/jump.cgi?ID=10434

Sportsman, S. (2005). Build a framework for conflict assessment. *Nursing Management, 36*(4), 32, 34–36, 38, 40.

Thomas, K. W., & Kilmann, R. H. (2007). *Conflict and conflict management.* Retrieved from http://www.kilmann.com/conflict.html

Tuckman, B. W. (2001). Developmental sequence in small groups. *Group Facilitation: A Research and Applications Journal, 3,* 66–80.

Zimmerman, P. G., & Jones, C. L. (2002). Negotiation. In P. G. Zimmerman (Ed.), *Nursing management secrets* (pp. 167–170). Philadelphia: Hanley & Belfus.

14

Current Theories of Change Management

BACKGROUND

- "The educator can help facilitate the initiation of, adoption of, and adaptation to change. Through leadership and participation in various activities such as committees, task forces, projects, and organizational strategic planning meetings, educators identify what changes should be made and can influence the necessary policy, procedures, or legislation to create change" (American Nurses Association, 2000, p. 9).
- Change is the process of altering or replacing existing knowledge, skills, attitudes, systems, policies, or procedures.
- Though change is a dynamic process that necessitates alterations in behavior and usually causes some conflict and resistance, it also can stimulate positive behaviors and attitudes and improve organizational outcomes and employee performance.
- Change is generally the result of identified problems in existing knowledge, skills, and systems; or of the need to change established ways of conducting business because of alterations in knowledge, technology, management, economics, or leadership.
- Problems are identified from many sources, including risk management data, quality improvement data, employee performance evaluations, and accreditation survey results.
- Change may be necessary due to changes in organizational structure or goals; accreditation criteria; legal mandates; or advances in diagnosis, treatment, and patient outcomes.

- Change at any level requires different behavior from the people involved.
- Skills needed to effect change include leadership, management, political savvy, analytical, interpersonal, system, business, and communication (Nickols, 2007; O'Shea, 2002).
- Systems change demands a "drastic shift in locus of control, accountability, expectations, performance, and measurement" (Malloch & Porter-O'Grady, 2006).
- The outcomes of change must be consistent with organizational mission, vision, and values.
- Because change is a constant in the healthcare environment, it is important to remember key points:
  - Employees will react differently to change, no matter how important or advantageous the change purports to be.
  - Basic needs will influence reaction to change, such as the need to be part of the change process, the need to be able to express oneself openly and honestly, and the need to feel that one has some control over the impact of change.
  - Change often results in loss (e.g., downsizing, changes in established routines) and employees may react with shock, anger, and resistance, and hopefully, ultimate acceptance.
  - Change must be managed realistically, without false hopes and expectations, yet with enthusiasm for the future.
  - It is important that management deal with the fears and concerns triggered by change in an honest manner (Monaghan, 2009; Team Technology, n.d.).

CHANGE THEORIES

- Below is a sample of both classic and current change theories. This list is not meant to be all-inclusive.
- *Lewin's Change Theory*
  - A three-step model based on the premise that behavior is a dynamic balance of forces working in opposition. Driving forces facilitate change by pushing employees in a desired direction, and inhibiting forces hamper change because they push employees in the opposite direction.
  - Step 1 is the process of altering behavior to "unfreeze," or agitate the status quo (equilibrium state). Step 1 is necessary if resistance is to be overcome and conformity achieved.
  - Step 2, "change", involves movement of the employees to a new level of equilibrium. It helps employees to view change from a new perspective, to work together to achieve desired outcomes of change, and to facilitate consistency among management and employees.
  - Step 3 is "refreezing," or attaining equilibrium with the newly desired behaviors. Step 3 occurs after change is implemented so that new behaviors and desired outcomes can be integrated into the organization (Lewin, 1951).
- *Lippitt's Seven-Step Change Theory*
  - Expands Lewin's theory to place additional emphasis on the role of the change agent.
  - Step 1: Diagnose the problem by examining all possible consequences, determining who will be affected by the change, identifying essential management personnel who will be responsible for fixing the problem, collecting data from those who will be affected by the change, and ensuring that those affected by the change will be committed to its success.
  - Step 2: Evaluate motivation and capability for change by identifying financial and human resources capacity and organizational structure.

- Step 3: Assess the change agent's motivation and resources, experience, stamina, and dedication.
- Step 4: Select progressive change objects by defining the change process and developing action plans and accompanying strategies.
- Step 5: Explain the role of the change agent to all involved employees (e.g., expert, facilitator, consultant) and ensure that expectations are clear.
- Step 6: Maintain change by facilitating feedback, enhancing communication, and coordinating the effects of change.
- Step 7: Gradually terminate the helping relationship of the change agent (Lippitt, Watson, & Wesley, 1958).
- Roger's Five-Stage Change Theory
  - Stage 1: Impart knowledge in terms of the reason for the change, how it will occur, and who will be involved.
  - Stage 2: Persuade employees to accept change by relaying essential information and note that attitudes, both favorable and unfavorable, are formed.
  - Stage 3: Decide whether to ultimately adopt the change by analyzing data and implementing a pilot study or trial of the new processes triggered by the change.
  - Stage 4: Implement the change on a more permanent or established basis as the organization evolves to accommodate the change.
  - Stage 5: Confirm adoption of the change by the employees responsible for and affected by the change (Rogers & Shoemaker, 1971).
- Spradley's Change Model
  - Consists of eight steps based on four concepts: system interdependence, homeostasis, opposing forces, and resistance.
    - Step 1: Identify the systems that trigger a need for change.
    - Step 2: Diagnose the problem that requires change.
    - Step 3: Assess all possible solutions to the problem.
    - Step 4: Select the best possible solution for change.
    - Step 5: Plan the change process.
    - Step 6: Implement the change process.
    - Step 7: Evaluate the effectiveness of the change process.
    - Step 8: Stabilize the behaviors desired and triggered by the change (Spradley, 1980).
- Appreciative Inquiry
  - Appreciative Inquiry (AI) takes an opposite approach. Rather than define a problem, AI looks at what works in an organization. Positive questions are asked to see potentials and possibilities to move toward.
  - There are four stages to the cycle of AI:
    - Discovery: Asking relevant stakeholders what is already positive in current practice: what is.
    - Dream: Through the use of imagination, create a clear vision for the future: what might be.
    - Design: Based on positive past achievements, identify the positive actions needed to reach the "dream": how to get there.
    - Destiny: Creating a climate for positive sustainable change: positive empowerment.
  - Central to AI's theory are five underlying principles:
    1. Constructionist Principle: People create their reality by how they view the world (organization).
    2. Poetic Principle: Organizations, like poems, are open to infinite interpretation.
    3. Simultaneity Principle: Change occurs as we talk about it.

4. Anticipatory Principle: Change is what we view as our future.
5. Positive Principle: Positive questions lead to positive images, which lead to positive energy and relationships (Cooperrider & Whitney, 2001).

- *Inspiration, Infrastructure, Education, Evidence (I_2E_2)*
  - A model for transforming the environment of care, specific to health care, integrating Appreciative Inquiry and advocating the engagement of groups and individuals to integrate change within the culture of an organization.
  - Four equal elements of the formula:
    1. Inspiration (I_1): Individuals are inspired by a clear vision and purposefulness: caring and healing relationships at the point of the care.
    2. Infrastructure (I_2): Provides the foundation and organization for change on three levels: strategic, operational, and tactical.
    3. Education (E_1): Promotes competence and personal commitment toward change through support to attain greatest capacity, leading to high role satisfaction.
    4. Evidence (E_2): Identifies that change has occurred and provides inspiration to begin the cycle again (Felgen, 2007).

CHANGE MANAGEMENT

- Change management is the process of making changes in a deliberate, planned, and systematic manner.
- Change management consists of theories, models, methods and techniques, tools, and skills.
- Knowledge of change management is drawn from numerous disciplines (e.g., psychology, business management, economics, engineering, organizational behavior).
- The goal of change management is to implement change efficiently for the benefit of the organization.
- Change has both content and process dimensions. Addressing underlying processes and effective communication of the change expectations leads to a successful change initiative.
- At the core of effective change are clearly defined outcomes of the proposed change, identified actions to attain the outcomes, and implementation of those actions (Monaghan, 2009; Nickols, 2007).

Creating a Climate for Effective Change

- Recognize that change is never easy and will be met with enthusiasm by some and resistance by others.
- Identify those who will be enthusiastic about the change (early adopters) and those will be resistors (laggers); involve them to build momentum and identify barriers, respectively.
- Collect and analyze data so that the need for change (and its consequences) can be articulated clearly.
- Give employees information honestly and allow them to ask questions and express concerns.
- Articulate the reasons for change, how it will affect employees, how it will benefit the organization, and the desired outcomes of the change process.
- Ensure leadership commitment so that leaders, in turn, can provide consistent information to their staff members (Jones, Aquirre, & Calderone, 2004; Monaghan, 2009; Nickols, 2007).

Resistance to Change

- Anticipate barriers to change, including components of organizational structure, and take action to remove them. Diffuse power groups and processes to prevent large barriers from systems and stakeholders (Porter-O'Grady & Malloch, 2003).
- Employees are resistant to change for a variety of reasons:
  - Fear of losing one's job, having to acquire new skills, and losing the ability to work effectively in a changed environment
  - Fear of losing one's unofficial power or influence
  - Failure to understand the reasons for change
  - Failure to understand how the change will benefit the workplace
  - Failure of management to involve affected employees in the change process
  - Failure of management to communicate effectively (e.g., not providing the reason for or full breadth of the change, limiting information to a few individuals, limiting methods used for communication)
  - Failure of management to relay facts about the change process honestly and realistically (Monaghan, 2009; Nickols, 2007)
- Change resistors must be identified, worked with, challenged, and placed in the midst of the change process so as not to impede the change process (Porter-O'Grady & Malloch, 2003).

The Process of Managing Change

- Identify the quality team members who have knowledge of and experience with change processes.
- Collect and analyze data regarding the need for change, desired outcomes, and impact on the organization and its employees.
- Pay close attention to the human aspects of change, dealing with such questions as: Will change result in downsizing? Will job requirements change? Will salaries be affected?
- Mobilize the CEO, administrative staff, and management; they must support the change process and speak with one voice about the process.
- Create ownership of the change process by including all levels of staff in the planning and implementation of the change process.
- Clearly and consistently communicate the action plan for change, emphasizing desired outcomes, why they are important, and the consequences if outcomes are not achieved.
- Include specific tasks and designate those responsible for achieving them. Set target dates for achievement in the action plan, and ensure this is communicated clearly.
- Offer training and continuing education relating to the change process, as well as for the acquisition of knowledge and skills necessary to achieve desired change outcomes.
- Address organizational culture and how the change will affect this culture.
- Incorporate symbolic and cultural norms into the communication process of change to aid in the adaptation to change.
- Deal with resistance calmly and objectively, explaining the consequences of failure to implement successful change.
- Recognize and reward the employees who contribute to the successful implementation of the change process.
- Change is a long-term process, so short-term goals must be identified to give stakeholders a sense of accomplishment.

- Alternate times of effort and action with periods of rest and celebration to reenergize for change, thereby decreasing change fatigue (Jones, Aquirre, & Calderone, 2004; Melnyk & Fineout-Overholt, 2005; Monaghan, 2009; Porter-O'Grady & Malloch, 2003).

Kotter's Heart of Change

- Moving away from strategy, structure, culture, and systems, the flow of see–feel–change is more powerful than analysis–think–change. The eight steps of successful change speak to people's feelings to change their behavior.
  - Step 1: Increase urgency; remove complacency, fear, and anger.
  - Step 2: Build the guiding team; choose the right people with the trust, commitment, and teamwork to get the job done.
  - Step 3: Get the vision right; provide clear direction that is bold and moving.
  - Step 4: Communicate for buy-in; share vision and strategies while addressing anger and anxiety to evoke faith in the vision.
  - Step 5: Empower action; remove barriers such as disempowering bosses, lack of information, wrong performance measure, and lack of self-confidence.
  - Step 6: Create the short-term wins; victories nourish faith, energize the change agents, defuse critics, and build momentum.
  - Step 7: Don't let up; build on momentum by keeping urgency up until the vision is a reality.
  - Step 8: Make change stick; embed a supportive culture for new way of operating (Kotter & Cohen, 2002).

REFERENCES

American Nurses Association. (2000). *Scope and standards of practice for nursing professional development.* Washington, DC: American Nurses Publishing.

Cooperrider, D. L., & Whitney, D. (2001). A positive revolution in change: Appreciative inquiry. Retrieved from http://appreciativeinquiry.case.edu/uploads/whatisai.pdf

Felgen, J. (2007). *I₂E₂: Leading lasting change.* Minneapolis, MN: Creative Healthcare Management.

Kotter, J. P., & Cohen, D. S. (2002). *The heart of change: Real-life stories of how people change their organizations.* Boston: Harvard Business School Press.

Jones, J., Aquirre, D., & Calderone, M. (2004). *10 principles of change management.* Retrieved from http://www.strategy-business.com/article/rr00006?pg=all

Lewin, K. (1951). *Field theory in social science.* New York: Harper & Row.

Lippitt, R., Watson, J., & Westley, B. (1958). *The dynamics of planned change.* New York: Harcourt, Brace & World.

Malloch, K., & Porter-O'Grady, T. (2006). *Introduction to evidence-based practice in nursing and health care.* Sudbury, MA: Jones & Bartlett.

Melnyk, B. M., & Fineout-Overholt, E. (2005). *Evidence-based practice in nursing & healthcare: A guide to best practice.* Philadelphia: Lippincott Williams & Wilkins.

Monaghan, H. M. (2009). Change & change agents. In S. L. Bruce (Ed.), *Core curriculum for staff development* (3rd ed., pp. 111–137). Pensacola, FL: National Nursing Staff Development Organization.

Nickols, F. (2007). *Change management 101: A primer.* Retrieved from http://www.nickols.us/change.pdf

O'Shea, K. L. (2002). *Staff development nursing secrets.* Philadelphia: Hanley & Belfus.

Porter-O'Grady, T., & Malloch, K. (2003). *Quantum leadership: A textbook of new leadership.* Sudbury, MA: Jones & Bartlett.

Rogers, E., & Shoemaker, F. (1971). *Communication of innovations: A cross-cultural approach.* New York: Free Press.

Spradley, B. W. (1980). Managing change creatively. *Journal of Nursing Administration, 52,* 32–37.

Team Technology. (n.d.). *Change management: Five basic principles, and how to apply them.* Retrieved from http://www.teamtechnology.co.uk/changemanagement.html

15

Resource Management

BACKGROUND

The American Nurses Association's (ANA, 2000, p. 21) Standard VII, Management and Resource Utilization, states "the nursing professional development educator considers factors related to safety; effectiveness; and cost in planning, delivering, and managing nursing professional development activities."

Team Management

- See Chapter 13's section on team building for further information.
- Regular feedback to teams is important for performance and to identify where the team fits into the "big picture."
- Clearly identify expectations and goals.
- Address conflicts as they arise; the longer a problem is allowed to fester within a team, the more energy and emotion it will take to resolve.
- Have the courage to accept responsibility; seek the truth, take risks, and stand up for what's right.

- Give the team the freedom to be successful.
- Give feedback on performance.
- Provide recognition for doing a job well (Cottrell, 2000).

Project Management

- See Chapter 16, Project Management.

Fiscal Management

- In the ANA *Standards of Professional Performance for Nursing Professional Development*, Standard VIII (quoted at beginning of chapter), one measurement criterion is: "The nursing professional development educator develops a financial plan sufficient to meet educational needs" (ANA, 2000, p. 21).
- Budgeting terms (see Chapter 10).
- Budgets can be defined by scope (e.g., project budget, department budget), purpose (e.g., supply budget, personnel budget), and time frame (e.g., monthly budget, annual budget; Smith, 2002).
- Determine department budget.
  - Look at past expenditures and revenue to assist with operating and capital budgets.
  - Operating budget: Used to account for revenue and expenses of day-to-day operations; includes income from goods and services, personnel costs, supplies and equipment.
  - Capital budget: Related to long-range planning for major cost items such as physical changes, major equipment and inventories; depreciation costs.
- Monitor budget.
  - Compare projected versus actual costs (variances) on a regular basis.
  - Document variances, both anticipated and unanticipated.
  - Implement cost-containment and reduction strategies as needed to keep costs within acceptable limits for volume.
  - Ensure all personnel are aware of costs (Avillion, Brunt, & Ferrell, 2007).
- Uses for a budget.
  - Document fiscal accountability of the professional development unit.
  - Identify and monitor trends in use of resources.
  - Evaluate educational activities and departmental functions from a financial viewpoint.
  - Project costs for new educational activities and initiatives.
  - Assess costs of current educational activities (Alspach, 1995).

Prioritization

- Be proactive rather than reactive in setting priorities.
- Base priorities on nursing service and organizational priorities.
- Planning is key to setting priorities and managing time.
  - Determine goals and rank by time: Time needed to complete planning and accomplish goals.
  - Identify plan: Include human and financial resources needed to accomplish goals.
  - Work the plan.
- Organize activities to facilitate achievement of goal or outcome.
  - Coordinate resources (people, equipment, and space).
  - Provide authority and communication.
- Delegate, use deadlines, and create a sense of urgency.
- Follow-up to ensure goal was met (Howard, 2009; Massello, 1998; Zimmermann, 2002).
- Alspach (1995) suggests basing priority on importance. To determine importance, consider:
  - High frequency (affects large number of staff)
  - High risk (harm to staff or patients if not done or not done correctly)
  - Problem-prone (produces problems for staff or patients)

Record Management

- See Chapter 12, Documentation and Records.

REFERENCES

Alspach, J. G. (1995). *The educational process in nursing staff development.* St. Louis, MO: Mosby.

American Nurses Association. (2000). *Scope and standards of practice for nursing professional development.* Washington, DC: American Nurses Publishing.

Avillion, A., Brunt, B., & Ferrell, M. J. (2007). *Nursing professional development review and resource manual.* Silver Spring, MD: American Nurses Credentialing Center.

Cottrell, D. (2000). *Listen up, leader! Pay attention, improve, and guide* (2nd ed.). Dallas, TX: Walk the Talk.

Howard, K. P. (2009). Role of the manager in staff development. In S. L. Bruce (Ed.), *Core curriculum for staff development* (3rd ed., pp. 451–474). Pensacola, FL: National Nursing Staff Development Organization.

Massello, D. J. (1998) Operations management: Administering the program. In K. J. Kelly-Thomas, *Clinical and nursing staff development: Current competence, future focus* (2nd ed., pp. 337–364). Philadelphia: Lippincott.

Smith, D. S. (2002). Managing budgets. In P. G. Zimmermann, *Nursing management secrets* (pp. 42–48). Philadelphia: Hanley & Belfus.

Zimmerman, P. G. (2002). Time management. In P. G. Zimmermann, *Nursing management secrets* (pp. 20–24). Philadelphia: Hanley & Belfus.

16

Project Management

BACKGROUND

- Project management entails planning, organizing, and managing resources to bring about successful completion of project goals and objectives.
- Characteristics of a project include:
  - Goal-oriented
  - Tasks that are connected and interrelated in a sequence
  - Limited duration
  - Unique and nonroutine
- Project management differs from program management because a program has no end. Program management improves performance on an ongoing program.
- Project management differs from priorities management, in which the goal is to separate the urgent from the truly important (Dobson, 1996).

PROJECT MANAGEMENT PROCESSES

- Initiate
  - Define project scope
  - Determine appropriate methods for completing project

- Plan and develop
  - Duration of tasks
  - Sequence of tasks
  - Resources
  - Costs
- Execute
  - Team leaders manage tasks within their expertise
  - Maintain accountability of team members
  - Track time and issues
  - Collaborate, collaborate, collaborate
- Monitor and control
  - Quality control: standards are met at each step of the project
  - Progress control: time schedules are met
  - Change control: changes are implemented with minimal delay
  - Issues management: time, fiscal, and resource challenges are addressed
- Close out the project
  - Resolve outstanding project items
  - Review control and change logs
  - Prepare project closure report
  - Review and update processes used by the project (Baker, Baker, & Campbell, 2003; Dobson, 1996).

PROJECT MANAGEMENT TOOLS

Gantt Chart

- A Gantt chart is a graphical representation of the duration of tasks against the progression of time.
- Tasks or activities are listed on the left side of the chart and dates are listed across the top. Activity duration is then indicated with a horizontal bar according to dates.
- A Gantt chart is a useful tool for planning and scheduling projects.
- A Gantt chart is helpful when monitoring a project's progress.

Cause and Effect Diagram

- A cause-and-effect diagram (also known as a "fishbone diagram") is a graphical technique for grouping people's ideas about the causes of a problem.
- Graphically illustrates the relationship between a given outcome and all the factors that influence the outcome (Arveson, 1996a).

RACI Diagram

- Describes the roles and responsibilities of various teams or people in delivering a project or operating a process.
- Processes or activities are listed down on the first column. Roles are listed along the top row.

- The cells are completed for who is **R**esponsible, **A**ccountable or must **A**pprove (may also use Supportive), who must be **C**onsulted and/or **I**nformed.
- It is especially useful in clarifying roles and responsibilities in cross-functional/departmental projects and processes (Value Based Management, 2010).

PERT Chart

- A PERT chart is a project management tool used to identify tasks and time estimates of complex projects.
- PERT stands for **P**rogram **E**valuation and **R**eview **T**echnique.
- The chart illustrates the activities that are performed sequentially and those performed in parallel.
- A PERT chart is beneficial for determining time requirements of complex projects (NetMBA, n.d.).

Flowchart

- Also known as a flow diagram, a flowchart uses graphic symbols to depict the nature and flow of steps in a process.
- Symbols used:
  - Oval: start point and end point
  - Box: an individual step or activity in the process
  - Diamond: a decision point in the process (e.g., yes/no, go/no go); each decision has a path to follow from the diamond
  - Circle: step is connected to another part or page of the flow chart and is indicated with a letter
  - Triangle: a place in the process where measurement occurs
- Benefits of flowcharts are:
  - Promote process understanding
  - Provide tools for training
  - Identify problem areas for improvement
  - Depict process relationships (Arveson, 1996b)

Project Management Resources

- Projects have three constraints: quality, money, and time.
- Quality requires clear outcome expectations of the project's scope. This is defined at the onset of the project.
- Money is the budget. Tap into resources in the finance department to assist with projecting costs.
- Time is managed through relationships and power.
- Because most projects are interdependent, it is important to develop collaborative relationships throughout the organization.
- "The real power to manage your project is not what others give you, it's what you make and what you take" (Dobson, 1996, p. 214).
- Achieve power through assertiveness, accomplishment, knowledge, relationships, initiative, people skills, communication, and understanding (Dobson, 1996).

REFERENCES

Arveson, P. (1996a). *Cause and effect diagram.* Retrieved from http://www.balancedscorecard.org/Portals/0/PDF/c-ediag.pdf

Arveson, P. (1996b). *Flowchart.* Retrieved from http://www.balancedscorecard.org/Portals/0/PDF/flowchrt.pdf

Baker, S., Baker, K., & Campbell, G. M. (2003). *The complete idiot's guide to project management* (3rd ed.). Indianapolis, IN: Alpha Book.

Dobson, M. (1996). *Practical project management: The secrets of managing any project on time and on budget.* Mission, KS: Skillpath Publications.

NetMBA (n.d.). *PERT.* Retrieved from http://www.netmba.com/operations/project/pert/

Value Based Management.net. (2010). *RACI model.* Retrieved from http://www.valuebasedmanagement.net/methods_raci.html

Wikipedia. (2010). *Project management.* Retrieved from http://en.wikipedia.org/wiki/Project_management

17

Consultation Process

BACKGROUND

- The nursing professional development educator acts in a formal or informal consultant role by:
  - Assisting with integration of new learning into the practice or educational environment
  - Serving as a resource in the design of needed educational experiences
  - Providing expertise for groups, departments, organizations, and other entities
  - Helping individuals and groups to define problems, identify internal and external educational resources, and select educational activities
  - Providing feedback to learners and the organization about the effectiveness of learning and the educational activity (American Nurses Association [ANA], 2000).
- *Consultation* is "a process of working with individuals or groups to help them solve work-related problems" (Norwood, 1998).
- *Internal consultant:* An employee within the organization who is in an advisory or support role.
- *External consultant:* An expert brought into an organization to guide, educate, or coordinate the effort of an organization through a contractually negotiated partnership for a designated time (Jackson, 2002).
- ANA Standards of Professional Performance related to the consultant role
  - *Standard IV—Collegiality:* "The nursing professional development educator interacts with, and contributes to the professional development of, peers and other health care providers as colleagues" (ANA, 2000, p. 18).

- *Standard VI—Collaboration:* "The nursing professional development educator collaborates with others in the practice of nursing professional development at the institutional, local, regional, state, national, or international levels" (ANA, 2000, p. 19).

Consultant Roles and Responsibilities

- Observer, fact-finder, expert: Analyzes a problem situation to determine the likely cause and suggests possible solutions.
- Change agent, facilitator: Helps with the implementation of behavioral, cognitive, affective, or organizational changes to resolve a problem.
- Educator, counselor: Offers education and clarifies situations based on problem analysis.
- Confidant, sounding board: Empowers clients and increases their self-sufficiency.
- Coach, motivator, mentor: Helps clients learn to use personal and professional resources more effectively (Norwood, 1998; Puetz & Shinn, 1997).

Consultant Skills

- Technical skills
  - Diagnostic skills
    - Ability to select and implement data-gathering approaches for assessment and evaluation
    - Broad understanding of and insight into multiple issues related to a problem (multicausality)
    - Ability to analyze and interpret data
    - Ability to synthesize information to draw conclusions about a problem's cause
  - Problem-solving skills
    - Ability to collaborate with clients in goal-setting, priority-setting, and task implementation
    - Ability to design, model, and implement a variety of problem-solving strategies
    - Ability to translate ideas into practice
    - Ability to mobilize resources and inspire clients
    - Political savvy
    - Risk-taking
- Human process skills
  - Communication skills
    - Effective verbal and nonverbal communication style
    - Ability to make formal written and verbal presentations
    - Ability to give and receive feedback
    - Ability to listen, question, clarify, and summarize
  - Interpersonal skills
    - Ability to create, maintain, and terminate relationships
    - Ability to manage a group effectively: maintain focus, manage conflicts, handle overt and hidden agendas
    - Ability to manage resistance or dependency
    - Negotiation (Grasnick, 2002; Norwood, 1998; Puetz & Shinn, 1997)

Contract Process

- A *contract* is an agreement that defines the purpose and goals of the relationship and delineates tasks, responsibilities, expectations, accountability, and the timeline for a project (Norwood, 1998).
- Components of a well-written contract include:
  - Statement of the problem and project goals
  - Services to be provided by the consultant: tasks, methods, products
  - Client responsibilities: tasks, supplies, resources, support they will provide
  - Timeline with specific start and end dates; also may include interim progress reports or meeting dates
  - Lines of authority, contact information, and communication expectations
  - Confidentiality limits on consultant access to people and information
  - Fees to be paid, expense reimbursement, and payment terms
  - Process for modifying or terminating contract, including description of penalties
  - Criteria and methods of evaluation and feedback
  - Signatures and dates of acceptance (Jackson, 2002; Norwood, 1998)

Consultation Process

- Gaining entry: Environmental scan, contract, physical entry, psychological entry
- Problem identification: Assess the situation, diagnose the problem, present analysis, redefine the current situation
- Action planning: Establish goals, evaluate possible interventions, provide recommendations, select course of action, develop an action plan, facilitate implementation
- Evaluation: Formative, summative, process, outcome
- Disengagement: Determine readiness, maintain change, manage psychodynamics, achieve closure (Norwood, 1998)

Questions Before Starting a Consultation

- Questions for the consultant to ask the client:
  - What results are you looking for?
  - What do you see as the main problem and what has been done so far to address the situation?
  - How long do you expect this will take?
  - What do you expect me to do for you?
  - What is the budget for the project?
  - Who is involved in the decision-making and who are the key players? (Jackson, 2002)
- Questions for the client to consider:
  - What do I want to happen as a result of the consultation?
  - What am I willing to do to accomplish this?
  - How much help do I want to accomplish this?
  - How much time can I devote to the project and when?
  - What resources can I provide?

- Questions for the consultant to consider:
  - What do I want from the consultation—fees, other rewards?
  - What am I willing to do to accomplish the goals of the consultation?
  - How much time am I willing to devote to the project and when?
  - What resources and support do I need from the client? (Norwood, 1998)

Preparing a Consultation Report

- Provide an overview of the problem: History, symptoms, challenges
- Summarize the assessment process: Purpose, data-gathering methodology, sources, theoretical framework
- Include data collection tools
- Describe observations and findings as well as the process for analysis
- Present conclusions and recommendations objectively
- Provide an implementation plan and timetable
- Summarize overall project process (Norwood, 1998; Puetz & Shinn, 1997)

Ethical and Legal Aspects of Consultation

- The ANA *Code of Ethics for Nurses* (ANA, 2001) provides a framework for ethical analysis and decision-making.
- Practice within limits of licensure, certification, education, and experience.
- Represent abilities accurately.
- Maintain boundaries between client interests and self-interest.
- Involve clients throughout the consultation process and respect their uniqueness.
- Demonstrate integrity and competence.
- Safeguard client welfare and confidentiality.
- Meet agreed-upon expectations.
- Provide documentation of process and outcomes (Norwood, 1998; Puetz & Shinn, 1997).

REFERENCES

American Nurses Association. (2000). *Scope and standards of practice for nursing professional development.* Washington, DC: American Nurses Publishing

American Nurses Association. (2001). *Code of ethics for nurses with interpretive statements.* Washington, DC: American Nurses Publishing.

Grasnick, L. L. (2002). Roles of the staff development educator. In K. L. O'Shea, *Staff development nursing secrets* (pp. 7–15). Philadelphia: Hanley & Belfus.

Jackson, M. J. (2002). Consultant. In B. E. Puetz & J. W. Aucoin (Eds.), *Conversations in nursing professional development* (pp. 79–87). Pensacola, FL: Pohl Publishing.

Norwood, S. L. (1998). *Nurses as consultants: Essential concepts and processes.* Menlo Park, CA: Addison-Wesley.

Puetz, L., & Shinn, L. J. (1997). *The nurse consultant's handbook.* New York: Springer.

Facilitation

BACKGROUND

- The nursing professional development educator acts as a facilitator by:
  - Assisting learners to identify learning needs and activities to meet those needs
  - Providing time for individuals to meet their educational needs or to access appropriate resources
  - Working with teams to brainstorm, problem-solve, and contribute to the strategic planning process
  - Serving as a role model for education and teamwork
  - Fostering a positive attitude about the benefits of lifelong learning (American Nurses Association [ANA], 2000).
- The purpose of *facilitation* is to help people accomplish goals and keep systems running smoothly (Grasnick, 2002).
- ANA Standards of Professional Performance related to the facilitator role include:
  - *Standard IV*—Collegiality: "The nursing professional development educator interacts with, and contributes to the professional development of, peers and other health care providers as colleagues" (ANA, 2000, p. 18).
  - *Standard VI*—Collaboration: "The nursing professional development educator collaborates with others in the practice of nursing professional development at the institutional, local, regional, state, national, or international levels" (ANA, 2000, p. 19).

Facilitator Roles and Responsibilities

- Involvement with learning activities
  - Work with learners to identify learning needs.
  - Plan activities to meet identified learning needs.
  - Collaborate within and across organization.
  - Create an environment that is conducive to learning: comfortable, interactive, and distraction-free.
  - Provide information and learning experiences using strategies that meet various learning needs and styles.
  - Help learners to access internal and external resources, serving as liaison if needed.
  - Provide feedback to learners (Brunt, 2007; Grasnick, 2002; Grey, 2002).
- Involvement with teams or projects
  - Educate team members about team processes such as quality improvement methodology, tools and techniques, and performance measurement and analysis.
  - Help the team establish and maintain effective working relationships and processes.
  - Coach the team in methods of data collection, data analysis, problem identification, and the development of improvement strategies.
  - Help the team prepare for formal presentations.
  - Work with the team to analyze the effectiveness of the team process.
  - Provide support and encouragement.
  - Use skills and knowledge of organizational processes to assist with removal of barriers or roadblocks (Brunt, 2007; Grasnick, 2002; Grey, 2002).

Developing Facilitation Skills

- Observe facilitation skills used by others or create a mentoring relationship with someone whose facilitation skills you admire.
- Learn as much as possible about the work environment (e.g., ways to get work done, obtain supplies, or locate other resources).
- Learn how to use library, audiovisual, and Internet resources.
- Identify people who are willing to serve as resources when needed, including support staff and individuals from other departments with relevant skills and expertise.
- Check with people often to find out how they are doing and whether they need help or support.
- Set limits and be honest with others about what you can realistically do to meet their needs.
- Document the assistance that you provide.
- Seek out opportunities to serve as facilitator to practice skills (Grasnick, 2002; Grey, 2002).

Common Facilitation Situations

- Interdisciplinary teams
  - An *interdisciplinary team* is a group composed of individuals with diverse yet complementary skills and perspectives, formed to collaborate to achieve a common purpose or goal.
  - May include representatives from clinical and nonclinical roles, leadership and staff positions, different disciplines, or other variations that bring individuals with the appropriate skills and knowledge to the table.

- The facilitator ensures balanced contributions within the group and keeps the group productive and focused on the goals (Clark, 2003; Grasnick, 2002; Norwood, 2003).
- Focus groups
  - A *focus group* is a group of individuals convened to share opinions as part of an interactive discussion about a product, service, concept, or idea.
  - A focus group consists of 4 to 12 people who participate in a 60- to 90-minute discussion.
  - The facilitator's role is to lead the discussion by asking open-ended questions that encourage dialogue related to specific objectives.
  - The facilitator uses skills to maintain the focus of the discussion, encourage balanced participation, and elicit honest opinions from the participants.
  - An observer is present to take notes and/or record the discussion with permission of the participants (Clark, 2003; Cooper, 2002; Kitchie, 2008; Yoder Wise, 1996).
- Strategic planning
  - *Strategic planning* is the process that an organization uses to determine direction, allocate resources, assign responsibilities, and set timelines to achieve realistic strategic goals.
  - The strategic planning process is applicable and shared at the unit, departmental, and institutional levels of an organization.
  - Strategic planning extends 3 to 5 years into the future.
  - The facilitator role in the strategic planning process may include educating the team about tools and techniques as well as maintaining the focus of the group's work.
  - Strategic planning process steps:
    - Conduct a SWOT (strengths, weaknesses, opportunities, threats) analysis.
    - Review/revise mission, vision, and values statements.
    - Identify strategic and operational goals.
    - Establish objectives and strategies to achieve goals.
    - Implement and evaluate effectiveness of strategies and achievement of objectives (Tomey, 2009).
  - An executive summary is a one- to two-page document that summarizes the key elements of the plan. It
    - Refreshes the mind of the reader concerning the project.
    - Provides a "5-minute" summary.
    - May become the only section of the plan that is read (Apeles, 2009).
- Meetings
  - *Meetings* are used for participative problem-solving, decision-making, coordination, information-sharing, and morale-building (Tomey, 2009).
  - Effective meetings have a defined purpose, are well-planned, and efficiently conducted to achieve the purpose.
  - Preparing for the meeting
    - Define the purpose/goal(s).
    - Select participants, location, date, and time.
    - Develop topics, presenters/responsible persons, attendees, outcomes, and time frames.
    - Distribute the agenda at least 24 hours in advance.
  - During the meeting
    - Start and end on time.
    - Follow the agenda.
    - Create a "parking lot" for side issues to be addressed later.
    - Evaluate meeting effectiveness.
  - After the meeting
    - Recap decisions and assignments.
    - Distribute minutes in a timely fashion (McNamara, n.d.; Tomey, 2009).

REFERENCES

American Nurses Association. (2000). *Scope and standards of practice for nursing professional development.* Washington, DC: American Nurses Publishing.

Apeles, N. C. (2009). Business and financial aspects of staff development. In S. Bruce (Ed.), *Core curriculum for staff development* (3rd ed.) Pensacola, FL: National Nursing Staff Development Organization.

Brunt, B. A. (2007). *Competencies for staff educators: Tools to evaluate and enhance nursing professional development.* Marblehead, MA: HCPro.

Clark, C. C. (2003). *Group leadership skills* (4th ed.). New York: Springer.

Cooper, D. C. (2002). Needs assessment. In K. L. O'Shea, *Staff development nursing secrets* (pp. 65–77). Philadelphia: Hanley & Belfus.

Cooper, D. C., & Bulmer, J. M. (2002). Staff development department management. In K. L. O'Shea, *Staff development nursing secrets* (pp. 47–57). Philadelphia: Hanley & Belfus.

Grasnick, L. L. (2002). Roles of the staff development educator. In K. L. O'Shea, *Staff development nursing secrets* (pp. 7–15). Philadelphia: Hanley & Belfus.

Grey, M. T. (2002). Change agent, facilitator, leader. In B. E. Puetz & J. W. Aucoin (Eds.), *Conversations in nursing professional development* (pp. 123–129). Pensacola, FL: Pohl Publishing.

Kitchie, S. (2008). Determinants of learning. In S. B. Bastable (Ed.), *Nurse as educator: Principles of teaching and learning for nursing practice* (3rd ed., pp. 93–145). Boston: Jones & Bartlett.

McNamara, C. (n.d.) *Basic guide to conducting effective meetings.* Retrieved from www.managementhelp.org/misc/mtgmgmnt.htm

Norwood, S. L. (2003). *Nursing consultation: A framework for working with communities.* Upper Saddle River, NJ: Pearson Education.

Tomey, A. M. (2009). *Guide to nursing management and leadership* (8th ed.). St. Louis, MO: Elsevier.

Yoder Wise, P. S. (1996). Learning needs assessment. In R. S. Abruzzese (Ed.), *Nursing staff development: Strategies for success* (2nd ed., pp. 188–207). St. Louis, MO: Mosby.

Coaching Process

BACKGROUND

- According to Standard IV of the *Standards for Professional Performance for Nursing Professional Development*, "The nursing professional development educator interacts with, and contributes to the professional development of, peers and other health care providers as colleagues" (American Nurses Association [ANA], 2000, p. 18).
- The coaching process is an effective tool to help others reach their full potential as members of the team.
- *Coaching* involves a partnership through which one offers support, provides learning opportunities, nurtures others to build on strengths, and acts to help them succeed (Kelly-Thomas, 1998).
- The nursing professional development educator may use coaching in situations of:
  - Remediation: Learner who is not meeting expectations; manager, preceptor, or others who are working with an employee requiring remediation
  - Career development: Staff and managers who are working toward career goals
  - Clinical advancement: Learner in transition (e.g., student to RN, LPN to BSN, staff nurse to charge nurse)

Attributes and Abilities of an Effective Coach

- Maturity
- Self-confidence
- Enthusiasm
- Sense of humor
- Humility
- Optimism
- Assertiveness
- Empathy
- Genuine interest and concern for others
- Tact
- Effective communication
- Open-mindedness
- Flexibility
- Goal orientation
- Resourcefulness
- Integrity (Ennis et al., 2005)

Coaching vs. Mentoring

- The terms "coaching" and "mentoring" are sometimes used interchangeably.
- *Mentoring* is a long-term partnership in which a more experienced individual partners with a less experienced individual to provide ongoing advice and counsel to guide career development (Zeus & Skiffington, 2002).
- *Coaching* is generally a short-term relationship involving an action plan to achieve specific goals for remediation or ongoing development.
- Some skills and traits are important to both coaching and mentoring relationships.

Core Principles of Coaching

- Focus on improvement of job performance rather than changing personality.
- Respect the dignity and worth of the individual.
- Focus on the current level of performance (Spangenberg, 2002).

Coaching for Remediation

- Analyze the facts and assess the importance of the performance concern before meeting with the person.
- Establish a one-to-one, private environment for discussion.
- Explain why a concern exists.
- Focus on behaviors rather than personal traits.
- Listen to the person's perspective.
- Mutually set realistic and attainable goals.

- Agree on actions to be taken (e.g., clear obstacles, set timelines, provide resources, adapt behaviors).
- Follow up to reflect, evaluate, and provide feedback.
- Celebrate success (Heathfield, 2010; Spangenberg, 2002).

Coaching for Career Development

- Combine coaching skills, role-modeling, and career management.
- Discuss career goals and pathways.
- Identify developmental needs and resources to enhance current skills and learn new skills.
- Clear obstacles and barriers to goal achievement.
- Provide support and encouragement.
- Celebrate success (Avillion, 2004; Zeus & Skiffington, 2002).

Coaching for Clinical Advancement

- Discuss needs to transform values, beliefs, and behaviors from past experience to current environment.
- Establish goals to meet identified needs.
- Provide resources and opportunities for training.
- Encourage growth by reinforcing strengths and removing barriers.
- Celebrate success.
- Encourage reflection.

REFERENCES

American Nurses Association. (2000). *Scope and standards of practice for nursing professional development.* Washington, DC: American Nurses Publishing.

Avillion, A. E. (2004). *A practical guide to staff development: Tools and techniques for effective education.* Marblehead, MA: HCPro.

Ennis, S., Goodman, R., Hodgetts, W., Hunt, J., Mansfield, R., Otto, J., & Stern, L. (2005). *Core competencies of the executive coach.* Retrieved from http://www.theexecutivecoachingforum.com/ECFCompetencyModel905.pdf

Heathfield, S. M. (2010). *Use employee coaching to improve performance.* About.com Retrieved from http://humanresources.about.com/od/glossaryc/g/coaching.htm

Kelly-Thomas, K. J. (1998). *Clinical and nursing staff development: Current competence, future focus* (2nd ed.). Philadelphia: Lippincott.

Spangenberg, S. L. (2002). When the problem is not an educational issue. In K. L. O'Shea (Ed.), *Staff development nursing secrets* (pp. 101–104). Philadelphia: Hanley & Belfus.

Zeus, P., & Skiffington, S. (2002). *The coaching at work toolkit: A complete guide to techniques and practices.* Sydney, AUS: McGraw Hill Australia.

Nursing Professional Development Quality Improvement

BACKGROUND

- "The nursing professional development educator systematically evaluates the quality and effectiveness of nursing professional development practice" (American Nurses Association [ANA], 2000, p. 16).
  - Identifies aspects of nursing professional development practice important for quality monitoring
  - Identifies indicators used to monitor quality and effectiveness of nursing professional development practice
  - Collects data to monitor quality and effectiveness of nursing professional development practice
  - Analyzes quality data to identify opportunities for improving nursing professional development practice
  - Evaluates learning activities
  - Formulates recommendations to improve nursing professional development practice or outcomes
  - Implements activities to enhance the quality of nursing professional development practice
  - Participates on intra- and interdisciplinary teams that evaluate professional development
  - Develops, implements, and evaluates policies and procedures to improve the quality of nursing professional development practice (ANA, 2000, p. 16)
- A *standard* is a statement that defines the expectations that must be met to ensure quality of care (Alspach, 1995).

- *Standards of nursing practice* are defined as "authoritative statements that describe a level of **care or performance** common to the profession of nursing by which the quality of nursing practice can be judged and measured" (ANA, 2000, p. 26).
- *Standards of professional performance* are "authoritative statements that describe a competent level of **behavior** in the professional role, including activities related to quality of care, performance appraisal, education, collegiality, ethics, collaboration, research, and resource utilization" (ANA, 2000, p. 26).
- *Quality improvement,* also called performance improvement or continuous quality improvement, refers to the continuous measurement and evaluation of a healthcare organization's functions and processes intended to achieve the desired outcomes of quality care and customer satisfaction (Joint Commission Resources, 2004; Webb, 2002).
- A *performance measure or indicator* is an objective, measurable, and achievable standard that is used to provide an indication of an organization's performance in relation to a specified process or outcome (Alspach, 1995; Joint Commission Resources, 2004; Webb, 2002).
- Performance indicators for nursing professional development are related to the orientation, inservice, and continuing education activities that assist nursing staff to develop, validate, and maintain the knowledge, attitude, and skills underlying nursing practice and quality patient care (Alspach, 1995).
- An *outcome measure* is "a measure that indicates the result of the performance (or nonperformance) of a function(s) or process(es)" (Joint Commission Resources, 2004, p. 136).
- Outcome measures for nursing professional development are related to:
  - Organizational mission, vision, and goals
  - Initial and ongoing competency assessment
  - Objective achievement and application to practice
  - Adherence with educational standards (e.g., American Nurses Credentialing Center, The Joint Commission)

Quality Improvement Models

- FOCUS—PDSA (or PDCA)
  - Find a process to improve
  - Organize a team
  - Clarify current knowledge of the process
  - Understand sources of process variation
  - Select the process improvement
  - Plan
  - Do
  - Study (or Check)
  - Act (Gloe, 1998; Joint Commission Resources, 2004; Tomey, 2009).
- PROCESS
  - Plan a purpose, team, and project scope
  - Research the current situation
  - Organize data and do a gap analysis
  - Create and try improvement
  - Evaluate trial results
  - Standardize the process
  - Start over (Joint Commission Resources, 2004)

- Critical path
  - Select and define a process
  - Form a team
  - Create the pathway
  - Implement the pathway (Joint Commission Resources, 2004)
- FADE
  - Focus on a strategic process to be improved
  - Analyze data to understand the current process or identify root causes of variation
  - Develop data-based action plans
  - Execute action plans with ongoing monitoring (Joint Commission Resources, 2004)

Roles in Quality Improvement

- Leaders facilitate interdisciplinary quality activities, build a culture of quality, communicate quality findings, and encourage others to be involved in quality improvement (Tomey, 2009).
- Managers monitor quality of care, facilitate quality data collection and analysis, keep current about quality-related standards and regulations, and facilitate ongoing quality improvement efforts (Tomey, 2009).
- Nursing professional development educators participate in organizational quality improvement efforts through competency assessments, provision of educational activities based on identified needs, evaluation of effectiveness of actions to improve performance, and communication of quality improvement results (Webb, 2002).
- Staff members participate in organizational quality improvement through involvement individually or in project teams, contributions to data collection and analysis, and implementation of improvements (Joint Commission Resources, 2004).
- Quality improvement specialists are responsible for coordinating quality improvement activities within an organization and coaching individuals and teams on quality improvement methods and tools. This role may be filled by one or more internal staff members or an external consultant (Joint Commission Resources, 2004).

Application to Nursing Professional Development

- Alspach (1995) identified three components of quality improvement in nursing professional development:
  1. Identification of standards that define quality in nursing professional development
  2. Monitoring of compliance with standards
  3. Institution of improvements in performance where indicated.
- Standards that define quality in nursing professional development include:
  - ANA *Scope and Standards for Nursing Professional Development* (2000)
  - Joint Commission Standards for Human Resources, Nursing, and others related to orientation, education, and competency assessment of nursing staff (Joint Commission Resources, 2009)
  - Specialty nursing organization standards related to education (e.g., Association of periOperative Registered Nurses, American Association of Critical-Care Nurses)
  - Baldrige National Quality Program *Education Criteria for Performance Excellence* (2009)

- Monitor compliance with standards
  - Determine performance indicators to be monitored.
  - Use benchmarking as a measure to compare performance with other departments, competitors or institutions.
  - Select data sources depending on indicators being measured. Possible sources include:
    - Educational records
    - Evaluation summaries
    - Test scores
    - Competency checklists
    - Results of surveys and questionnaires
    - Chart audits or reviews
    - Observation
    - Peer review
  - Use data collection tools that are clear and simple.
  - Analyze data using statistical and nonstatistical tools and techniques to identify areas for improvement.
    - Statistical tools: Run charts, histograms, control charts, scatter diagrams, Pareto charts, decision matrix, bar graphs
    - Nonstatistical tools: Flowcharts, fishbone diagrams, cause-and-effect diagrams (Alspach, 1995; Gloe, 1998; Joint Commission Resources, 2004; Katz, 1996; Tomey, 2009; Webb, 2002)
- Institute performance improvements where indicated.
  - Determine recommendations to improve practice or outcomes.
  - Use defined process to implement recommendations (e.g., pilot process, PDSA cycle).
  - Allow time for change in behavior to occur.
  - Continue monitoring to hold the gains, using the same performance indicators and data collection tools used previously (Joint Commission Resources, 2004; Webb, 2002).

Example of Quality Improvement in Nursing Professional Development

- Identify standard of quality in nursing professional development.
  - Standard of Practice IV: Planning—"The nursing professional development educator identifies and collaborates with content experts to develop activities to facilitate learners' achievement of the educational objectives" (ANA, 2000, p. 13).
  - Measurement criterion—"The content is developed with input from the target audience" (ANA, 2000, p. 14).
- Monitor compliance with standards.
  - Determine the performance indicator—representatives of the target audience (learners) participate in planning the educational activity.
  - Select data sources—list of educational activities for 6-month period, planning meeting minutes, e-mails of planning committee, course evaluation summaries.
  - Gather data—for example, a total of 14 educational activities during 6-month period, written and electronic documentation shows that 12 of 14 activities included at least one representative of target audience in planning group; two activities without target audience representation were specialty grand rounds; one course's evaluation summary requested expansion of topic content.

- Analyze data—opportunity for improvement, specifically with group planning grand rounds and course content change for identified course.
- Institute improvements in performance—work with planning group leadership to develop plan for involvement of target audience representative; incorporate change in course content; assess need for policy development or revision and time needed for course revisions.
- Gather data again in 6 months.

Departmental Structure

- Placement of the nursing professional development staff and work unit within the organizational structure influences and is influenced by the unit's responsibilities and scope.
- Other factors that affect the responsibilities and scope of nursing professional development within an organization include size of organization, number of employees, organizational mission, and type of institution (Puetz & Aucoin, 2002).
- Nursing professional development may be structured in one of the following ways, each of which has quality advantages and disadvantages:
  - Institution-wide: Centralized department responsible for staff education in multiple departments throughout the institution
    - Advantages: Coordination of resources and required programming, uniform implementation of standards, comprehensive orientation, consistent content and teaching methods, efficient use of staff and support services
    - Disadvantages: Centralized decision-making may be unaware of or unresponsive to unit needs, lack of coordination or identity with specific areas, potential loss of autonomy or clinical skills of educators
  - Nursing department: Department or division responsible for education of nursing department staff; may organize all nursing professional development functions centrally or manage some centrally with others at the specialty or unit level
    - Advantages: Easier identification of unit educational needs, flexibility and timeliness in providing educational activities, educational leadership and involvement in departments, increased opportunity for feedback, educators seen as clinical experts
    - Disadvantages: Duplication of education and staff effort, inconsistent education content and teaching methods, ineffective or inefficient coordination, lack of support services, educators may be used for service
  - Combination of institution-wide and nursing department: Uses portion of both centralized and decentralized structures to manage and deliver education
    - Advantages: Identification of and timely response to unit needs, use of clinical experts for unit-based educational activities, coordination reduces duplication and inappropriate use of resources, availability of support services, collegial support for educators
    - Disadvantages: Potential increased staffing and costs of managing both structures, educators may lose sight of overall staff development goals (Alspach, 1995; Brunt, 1998; Hood, 2002)
  - Cooperative or consortium: Collaborative effort between two or more organizations (e.g., hospital, college or university, long-term-care facility) where professional development educators share responsibilities for staff education; may include nursing and non-nursing roles
    - Advantage: Ability to provide more and higher quality programs at a lower cost
    - Disadvantage: Requires collaboration and shared planning for consensus on products, facilities, and resources (Brunt, 1998)

REFERENCES

Alspach, J. G. (1995). *The educational process in nursing staff development.* St. Louis, MO: Mosby.

American Nurses Association. (2000). *Scope and standards of practice for nursing professional development.* Washington, DC: American Nurses Publishing.

Baldrige National Quality Program. (2009). *Education criteria for performance excellence.* Gaithersburg, MD: Author.

Brunt, B. A. (1998). Structure and process: New models of nursing and clinical staff development. In K. J. Kelly-Thomas, *Clinical and nursing staff development: Current competence, future focus* (2nd ed., pp. 25–53). Philadelphia: Lippincott.

Gloe, D. (1998). Quality management: A staff development tradition. In K. J. Kelly-Thomas, *Clinical and nursing staff development: Current competence, future focus* (2nd ed., pp. 301–336). Philadelphia: Lippincott.

Hood, A. W. (2002). Factors that affect the educator's role. In K. L. O'Shea, *Staff development nursing secrets* (pp. 17–25). Philadelphia: Hanley & Belfus.

Joint Commission Resources. (2004). *Cost-effective performance improvement in hospitals.* Oakbrook Terrace, IL: Author.

Joint Commission Resources. (2009). *Joint commission requirements.* Retrieved from http://www.jointcommission.org/Standards/Requirements/

Katz, J. M. (1996). Managing the dual dimensions of quality. In R. S. Abruzzese (Ed.), *Nursing staff development: Strategies for success* (2nd ed., pp.302–325). St. Louis, MO: Mosby.

Puetz, B. E., & Aucoin, J. A. (2002). *Conversations in nursing professional development.* Pensacola, FL: Pohl Publishing.

Tomey, A. M. (2009). *Nursing management and leadership* (8th ed.). St. Louis, MO: Elsevier.

Webb, D. G. (2002). Performance improvement. In B. E. Puetz & J. W. Aucoin (Eds.), *Conversations in nursing professional development* (pp. 255–260). Pensacola, FL: Pohl Publishing.

21

Research Process

BACKGROUND

- Standard VII of the American Nurses Association's *Standards for Nursing Professional Development*—Research: "The nursing professional development educator participates in and uses evidence-based research to identify strategies for improving professional development activities, nursing practice, and patient outcomes" (ANA, 2000, p. 20)
- Research competencies for the nursing professional development educator identified by Brunt (2007):
  - Supports integration of research into practice
  - Incorporates research findings from a variety of disciplines into programs
  - Accesses resources needed to facilitate research
  - Develops and conducts research

IDENTIFY THE PROBLEM

- Cannot be general; must be narrowed to reflect a specific problem.
- Guides the research process.
- Must be clearly stated before research can begin.
- Requires considerable thought, imagination, creativity.
- Must be significant, researchable, and feasible.
- Needs to be an area of interest (Polit & Beck, 2007; Wood & Ross-Kerr, 2006).

Sources of Research Problems

- Experience: immediate needs that are relevant and interesting
- Nursing literature: regular reading of research literature can identify areas of interest, problems, or inconsistencies that need to be addressed
- Theory: test applicability to nursing or nursing education
- Ideas from external sources: a direct suggestion from faculty, employer, or funding agencies (Polit & Beck, 2007)

Searching the Literature

- May use librarian for assistance.
- Access online databases for nursing, medical, and healthcare information (e.g., PubMed, Medscape, Nursing Center) as well as non-healthcare resources if applicable to the topic area.
- Helps researcher become familiar with current knowledge in area of interest.
- Helps refine the research problem.
- Determines if there are similar studies that could be replicated or refined.
- May reveal previous methods that have proven useful in similar circumstances.
- Can solidify need for or significance of research in problem area.
- Using original (i.e., primary) sources rather than secondary sources.
- Needs to be comprehensive and include all relevant literature (Wood & Ross-Kerr, 2006).

Evaluating Research Articles

- Using the ASK (Applicability, Science, Knowledge) model
- *Applicability*
  - Is this study relevant to practice?
  - Do the findings suggest that the interventions tested made statistical or clinical improvements to practice?
  - Does the benefit to the subject outweigh the risk of implementation?
  - Is the change cost-effective in terms of human and material resources?
  - Is the potential outcome for the subject or organization worth the effort to implement the change?

- *Science*
  - The science is evaluated using standard criteria regardless of the practice area
  - "SPRMA" or "SPRTMA"—acronyms to help reviewers remember the key components of research
    - **S** – Statement of the problem
    - **P** – Purpose
    - **R** – Research question
    - **T** – Theoretical framework
    - **M** – Methodology
    - **A** – Analysis
- *Knowledge*
  - Do the results fit the existing knowledge base?
  - Do the research findings have meaning to the reader's knowledge base?
  - Why wouldn't or shouldn't I use this idea? (Dittman, 2002)

Research Aims, Questions, Hypotheses, and Operational Definitions

- *Aim* outlines what the study is trying to achieve.
- Research *questions* narrow the original problem to a more concise statement that is measurable.
- *Hypothesis* is a statement about a relationship between two or more variables and predicts an expected outcome.
- The *independent variable* is the variable that the researcher chooses to control.
- The *dependent variable* is the variable that is affected by the independent variable.
- *Operational definitions* state the meanings of terms and how the terms will be measured (Polit & Beck, 2007).

RESEARCH DESIGN

- The research design guides the researcher in an organized fashion throughout the study.
- Strategies for sampling, data collection, and analysis of findings are determined by selection of a research design.
- A pilot study may be used to test the reliability and validity of data collection tools, or allow the researcher to practice research skills, such as interviewing techniques.
- Provides a plan or blueprint to answer the research question.
- Internal and external validity as concepts basic to the issue of control.
  - *Internal validity:* The extent to which the results of the study can actually be attributed to the action of the independent variable and not something else
  - *External validity:* the degree to which the findings of the study are generalizable to the target population (Wood & Ross-Kerr, 2006)

Types of Research Designs

- Descriptive: Results in a description of the data, whether in words, pictures, charts, or tables, and whether the data analysis shows statistical or merely descriptive relationships

- Experimental: Results in inferences drawn from the data that explain the relationships between the variables
- Types of quantitative research designs
  - *Experimental:* Subjects are randomly assigned to treatment or control group where the researcher manipulates the *independent variable* (the intervention, treatment, or condition introduced) and measures the effect achieved by the independent variable on the *dependent variable*
  - *Quasi-experimental:* Experimental treatment with a nonequivalent control group or no randomization, such as data collection before and after a treatment, or a time series design in which data are obtained from one group at several points before and after the treatment
  - *Nonexperimental:* Researcher collects data without making changes or introducing an intervention
    - Exploratory: Provides in-depth exploration of a single process or variable
    - Descriptive: Identifies characteristics of a specific population at one point
    - Retrospective: Ex post facto studies in which the researcher identifies a current phenomenon and collects data from the past in an attempt to identify possible causal factors
    - Prospective: Type of longitudinal study in which a group of subjects with a condition at present is followed over time to identify outcomes
    - Correlational: Used to examine the type and degree of the relationship between two variables
    - Case control studies: Descriptive study of a group of subjects with a condition compared to a group of subjects without the condition
- Surveys look at variables in a specific population or groups through self-report information.
- Needs assessments provide basis for development of a policy or program.
- Methodology studies examine the validity and reliability of instruments (Parker, 2009).

DATA COLLECTION

Sampling Techniques

- *Probability sampling* reflects the use of random selection, with every member of the target population having an equal chance of being included in the sample; includes simple random sampling, stratified random sampling, and cluster sampling.
  - *Simple random sampling* uses a table of random numbers to ensure that each unit in the population has an equal and independent chance of being selected.
  - *Stratified random sampling* divides the population into strata based on the sample criteria, then draws a predetermined number from each group using random sampling techniques.
  - *Cluster sampling* involves repeated random sampling progressing from large to small units over two or more stages (e.g., choosing a selection of samples from home health agencies, then selecting a sample of nurse case managers in home health agencies).
- *Nonprobability (convenience) sampling* reflects selection without the use of random selection; includes convenience, quota, systematic, and network sampling.
  - *Convenience sampling:* A minimum number of subjects or time frame is determined and everyone who meets the criteria is invited to participate.

- *Quota sampling:* Criteria to divide the sample into groups are identified, and then convenience sampling is used to fill the quota in each group.
- *Systematic sampling:* Selection of every *nth* number of the available population, after beginning with a random start.
- *Network sampling:* An individual or group meeting the sample criteria is identified, and the first and each subsequent member of the sample are asked to provide names of other individuals meeting the sample criteria (Wood & Ross-Kerr, 2006).

Data Collection Techniques

- Data collection methods are based on the hypothesis, research design, and characteristics of the population being studied.
- Methods of data collection:
  - Observation
  - Questionnaires
  - Interviews
  - Available data
  - Physiological measures
- Instruments must be reliable and valid.
  - Reliability addresses consistency, stability, repeatability, dependability, predictability, and accuracy of the measurement.
  - Validity is concerned with how well the instrument measures what it is intended to measure (Parker, 2009; Polit & Beck, 2007; Wood & Ross-Kerr, 2006).

DATA ANALYSIS

- Purpose of data analysis "is to reduce, organize, and give meaning to data" (Parker, 2009, p. 501).
- Types of data:
  - Qualitative: Verbal, narrative pieces of information
  - Quantitative: Numerical information
- Four levels of quantitative measurement:
  - *Nominal:* Mutually exclusive variables are organized into categories that cannot be compared, such as gender or marital status
  - *Ordinal:* Categories are ranked by the interval between rankings and are not necessarily equal, such as levels of pain or educational levels
  - *Interval:* Equal numerical distances exist between variables, such as a 1–5 rating scale
  - *Ratio:* Highest measurement form expressing a continuum of values with an absolute zero, such as weight
- Statistical analysis is used for quantitative data.
  - *Descriptive statistics* describe data (e.g., frequency, mean, range, standard deviation, correlation)
  - *Inferential statistics* draw conclusions about population from relationships between variables (e.g., *t* test, analysis of variance, chi-square, regression)

- Existence: Does a relationship exist between variables?
- Magnitude: What is the strength of the relationship between variables?
- Nature: What type of relationship exists between variables?

- Data analysis can be about one (univariate), two (bivariate), or three or more (multivariate) variables.
- Data analysis is done for different purposes.
  - Data cleaning: Done before analysis to find errors in data entry
  - Sample description: Summarize sample attributes (i.e., demographics)
  - Assessment of bias: Identify systematic biases (e.g., characteristics of volunteer subjects)
  - Evaluation of measurement tools: Analysis of validity and reliability of instruments
  - Evaluation of the need for transformations: How to handle missing values
  - Addressing research questions
- When addressing research question(s), statistical tests reject or accept the null (no difference) hypothesis.
- Type I error: Determine a difference exists when in actuality no difference exists.
  - Control for Type I error with "level of significance" (e.g., 0.05 or 0.01 levels of significance)
- Type II error: Determine no difference exists when in actuality a difference does exist.
  - Control for Type II error through power analysis (e.g., reaching sample size to a power of 0.80; typically determined prior to data collection)
- Biostatisticians can be helpful in determining sample size needed and identifying statistical tests to be done.
- Generally, a computer software program is used to analyze data.
- Create and follow a data analysis plan to decrease measurement error.
- Data analysis occurs during data collection to clean data, assess bias, evaluate measurement tools, and address missing data problems.

Interpreting the Results

- Explore significance of results.
- Describe limitations.
- Formulate conclusions.
- Identify implications and recommendations for future studies.
- Communicate findings.
  - Descriptive statistics—narrative, graph(s), table(s)
  - Inferential statistics—narrative, table(s)
  - Report to stakeholders
  - Poster or paper presentations
  - Manuscript (Parker, 2009; Polit, 1996)

INSTITUTIONAL REVIEW BOARD (IRB)

- Prior to implementation, all research should be approved by a qualified review board to ensure patient protection and ethical integrity.
- The IRB is a group that approves, monitors, and reviews biomedical research involving human subjects.

- Assures "that appropriate steps are taken to protect the rights and welfare of humans participating as subjects in research" (Food and Drug Administration, 2009).
- Issues of particular concern to the IRB are ethics, informed consent, confidentiality, and patient safety.
- Educational research typically falls under an expedited review.
- An expedited review can be done by the chair of the IRB or a designee rather than full IRB membership.
- Expedited review is used for research when:
  - The research poses minimal risk to the subject.
  - Data collection is noninvasive.
  - Data was or will be collected normally as a part of clinical practice (e.g., medical diagnosis).
  - Research is on individual or group characteristics or behavior (e.g., cognition, motivation, social behavior).
  - Research uses survey, interview, oral history, focus group, program evaluation, human factors evaluation, or quality assurance methodologies (Health and Human Services, 1998).

Elements of Informed Consent

- Purpose and procedures of the research
- Description of subject selection process
- Description of potential risks, discomfort, and/or benefits to the subject or others
- Statement of how confidentiality of records will be maintained
- Compensation, if any, is discussed
- Alternative procedures, if any, are disclosed
- Right to refuse to participate or withdraw from study without penalty is assured
- The IRB may waive some or all of the informed consent process when:
  - No more than minimal risk to subject is involved,
  - Absence of informed consent does not adversely affect the subjects' rights and welfare,
  - The research could not be carried out without the waiver, and
  - When possible, the subjects are provided with information after participation (Health and Human Services, n.d.).

REFERENCES

American Nurses Association. (2000). *Scope and standards of practice for nursing professional development.* Washington, DC: American Nurses Publishing.

Brunt, B. A. (2007). *Competencies for staff educators: Tools to evaluate and enhance nursing professional development.* Marblehead, MA: HCPro.

Dittman, P. W. (2002). Researcher. In B. E. Puetz & J. W. Aucoin (Eds.), *Conversations in nursing professional development* (pp. 89–101). Pensacola, FL: Pohl Publishing.

Food and Drug Administration. (2009). *Running clinical trials: Frequently asked questions.* Retrieved from http://www.fda.gov/ScienceResearch/SpecialTopics/RunningClinicalTrials/GuidancesInformationSheetsandNotices/ucm115632.htm

Health and Human Services. (1998). *Categories of research that may be reviewed by the Institutional Review Board (IRB) through an expedited review.* Retrieved from http://www.hhs.gov/ohrp/humansubjects/guidance/expedited98.htm

Health and Human Services. (n.d.). Chapter III: Basic IRB review. In *Institutional Review Board guidebook.* Retrieved from http://www.hhs.gov/ohrp/irb/irb_chapter3.htm#e2

Parker, E. B. (2009). Researcher role of the nursing professional development educator. In S. L. Bruce (Ed.), *Core curriculum for staff development* (3rd ed., pp. 487–509). Pensacola, FL: National Nursing Staff Development Organization.

Polit, D. F. (1996). *Data analysis & statistics for nursing research.* Stamford, CT: Appleton & Lange.

Polit, D. F., & Beck, C. T. (2007). *Nursing research: Generating and assessing evidence for nursing practice.* Philadelphia : Lippincott Williams & Wilkins.

Wood, P. J., & Ross-Kerr, J. C. (2006). *Basic steps in planning nursing research: From question to proposal* (6th ed.). Sudbury, MA: Jones & Bartlett.

22

Evidence-Based Practice

BACKGROUND

- According to a measurement criterion for Standard of Professional Performance VII: Research (American Nurses Association [ANA], 2000), "The nursing professional development educator uses available evidence, including research data, in the educational process" (p. 20).
- *Evidence-based practice* is "a practice that involves making clinical decisions on the best available evidence, with an emphasis on evidence from disciplined research" (Polit & Beck, 2010).
- Evidence-based practice has also been described as a problem-solving approach that addresses a question by integrating:
  - A systematic search for and appraisal of the most relevant evidence
  - One's own clinical expertise
  - Patient preferences and values (Melnyk & Fineout-Overholt, 2005)
- Just as nurses are expected to use evidence-based practice in clinical practice, nursing professional development educators need to base their practice on current evidence (Brunt, 2007).
- The nursing professional development educator incorporates evidence-based practice through:
  - Integration of evidence-based practice into their practice
  - Facilitation of evidence-based practice as part of their role
  - Application of evidence-based practice within the educational process

Steps of Evidence-Based Practice

- Step 1: Formulate the burning clinical question in the PICO format: **P**atient population, **I**ntervention of interest, **C**omparison intervention or status, and **O**utcome.
- Step 2: Search for best evidence from a hierarchy of evidence.
- Step 3: Conduct a critical review of the evidence.
- Step 4: Integrate the evidence with the provider's expertise, assessment of the patient, available resources, and the patient's preferences.
- Step 5: Evaluate the effectiveness of the evidenced-based intervention in meeting the desired outcome (Melnyk & Fineout-Overholt, 2005).

Rating System for Hierarchy of Evidence

- Level I: Evidence from a systematic review or meta-analysis of relevant randomized controlled trials or evidence-based guidelines based on such reviews
- Level II: Evidence from at least one well-designed randomized controlled trial
- Level III: Evidence obtained from well-designed controlled trials without randomization
- Level IV: Evidence from well-designed case-control and cohort studies
- Level V: Evidence from systematic reviews of descriptive and qualitative studies
- Level VI: Evidence from a single descriptive or qualitative study
- Level VII: Evidence from the opinion of authorities and/or expert committees (Melnyk & Fineout-Overholt, 2005; Polit & Beck, 2010)

See Chapter 6, Issues and Trends, for additional information about evidence-based practice and sources of evidence.

Advantages to Evidence-Based Practice in Nursing Professional Development

- Provides high-quality, cost-effective educational services from a knowledge and/or evidence base
- Bridges the gap between theory and practice
- Supports the need for and stimulates interest in staff development research
- Improves staff development services to improve learners' job performance
- Enhances use of evidence in communication among departments
- Increases job satisfaction among nursing professional development educators (Avillion, 2007)

Barriers to Evidence-Based Practice in Nursing Professional Development

- Shortage of research in the field of nursing professional development
- Lack of knowledge about the research process
- Lack of time for reading and evaluating research
- Lack of time for participating in the research process
- Staff resistance within the education department as well as by learners
- Cost to conduct research, analyze data, and implement practice changes (Avillion, 2007).

Integration of Evidence-Based Practice Into NPD Practice

- Dissemination of current evidence-based findings through educational activities.
  - Base educational programs and competencies on current evidence when possible.
  - Discuss evidence and its applicability to practice in didactic or experiential learning activities.
  - Conduct periodic reviews and update ongoing educational activities to incorporate current evidence.
  - Include examples of evidence-based practice in the orientation process.
- Review course content annually to ensure it is current with the evidence.
- Maintain print or electronic files as you find evidence-based literature relevant to your work.
- Use current evidence in the development of practice documents such as policies, procedures, standards, and guidelines.
- Submit practice documents for periodic review to incorporate the latest evidence (Grasmick, 2002; Krugman, 2002).

Facilitation of Evidence-Based Practice as Part of the NPD Role

- Provide leadership in departmental activities that promote the use of evidence-based practice.
  - Participate in research committees or councils.
  - Collaborate with management, advanced practice nurses, and nursing staff to initiate and support evidence-based practice activities.
  - Ensure that the facility's medical library subscribes to research and evidence-based resources relevant to nursing.
  - Foster preceptor activities that promote valuing of evidence-based practice.
- Implement strategies that expose learners to sources of evidence.
  - Post relevant evidence-based articles for staff to read.
  - Establish a journal club for discussion of evidence-based articles.
  - Invite colleagues to present evidence-based practice projects to staff.
- Offer a course on evidence-based practice (Melnyk & Fineoult-Overholt, 2005; Grasmick, 2002; Krugman, 2002).

Application of Evidence-Based Practice in the Educational Process

- Incorporate current evidence about educational process or strategies, educator expertise, and learner behaviors (e.g., teaching methodologies, learning outcomes, testing methods) into educational activities.
- Apply the steps of evidence-based practice to the educational environment.
  - Question teaching strategies or educational practices.
  - Search for best evidence.
  - Critically review the evidence to determine if it applies in this situation.
  - Use the evidence to plan teaching strategies, evaluation methods, etc.
  - Evaluate the effectiveness of methods (Melnyk & Fineoult-Overholt, 2005; Krugman, 2002).

REFERENCES

American Nurses Association. (2000). *Scope and standards of practice for nursing professional development.* Washington, DC: American Nurses Publishing.

Avillion, A. E. (2007). *Evidence-based staff development: Strategies to create, measure, and refine your program.* Marblehead, MA: HCPro.

Brunt, B. A. (2007). *Competencies for staff educators: Tools to evaluate and enhance nursing professional development.* Marblehead, MA: HCPro.

Grasmick, L. L. (2002). Roles of the staff development educator. In K. L. O'Shea (Ed.), *Staff development nursing secrets* (pp. 7–15). Philadelphia: Hanley & Belfus.

Krugman, M. (2002). Evidence-based practice. In B. E. Puetz & J. W. Aucoin (Eds.), *Conversations in nursing professional development* (pp. 349–364). Pensacola, FL: Pohl Publishing.

Melnyk, B. M., & Fineout-Overholt, E. (2005). *Evidence-based practice in nursing and healthcare: A guide to best practice.* Philadelphia: Lippincott Williams & Wilkins.

Polit, D. F., & Beck, C. T. (2010). *Essentials of nursing research: Appraising evidence for nursing practice* (7th ed.). Philadelphia: Wolters Kluwer/Lippincott Williams & Wilkins.

23

Informatics

INFORMATION MANAGEMENT

- Computer skills are essential for the nursing professional development educator.
- The basic software programs on a personal computer include word processing, spreadsheet, and graphics presentation software (e.g., Microsoft Office, Lotus Suite, Apple iWork).
- Word processing enables development of handouts, notes, and documents.
- Spreadsheets are used to manage education budget and maintain educational records.
- Graphics presentation software (e.g., Microsoft PowerPoint, Apple Keynote) provides capability for electronic slides with graphics, text, and video and sound clips.
- A desktop publishing program (e.g., Microsoft Publisher, Apple Pages) provides preformatted newsletters, brochures, letters, and labels, allowing for design of sophisticated fliers to market educational activities.
- Communication is enhanced via e-mail programs, intranet, and Internet access.
- Most e-mail programs have calendar and appointment features. Use of this technology increases efficiency.
- The Internet provides access to search engines (e.g., Bing, Google, Yahoo!) and databases for nursing, medical, and healthcare information (e.g., PubMed, Medscape, Nursing Center).
- The nursing professional development educator develops skills for use of these programs via classes, which may be offered by the organization, and on-the-job experience (Bowman, 2002).

- Organization-specific information is exchanged via an intranet. Items on an intranet may include hospital newsletters, policies and procedures, laboratory manual, and medical references. Employees are given access via user names and passwords.
- Other hospital systems also employ user names and passwords (e.g., medication and supply access, glucose monitoring devices, clinical information systems, e-mail, access to medical references).
- One's role within the organization determines the level of access to these systems.
- The information technology (IT) department is the typical contact for assigning user names and passwords, as well as troubleshooting and resetting forgotten passwords.

INFORMATION PROCESSING

Collecting Data

- Data can be collected via paper, scannable forms, computer, or the Web.
- Data from interviews or focus groups need to be transcribed into electronic form for ease of analysis.
- The most common form of data collection is on paper from sources such as surveys, interviews, questionnaires, tests, chart audits, and course evaluations.
- Paper data need to be collated, organized, and presented in a fashion to allow interpretation and spot trends.
- Data entry by hand requires time, cost, and "cleaning" for error identification.
- Scannable forms are paper-based but remove the data entry component. Design can include the familiar "bubble" and fill-in fields. Hardware and software are needed to read the forms and convert to electronic data.
- Computerized tests allow data to be scored, collated, and analyzed more readily than paper tests.
- Web-based surveys
  - Are less costly than paper surveys and questionnaires because reproduction, mailing, and data entry expenses are eliminated.
  - Data from Web-based surveys are easily imported into spreadsheet or statistical software.
  - Requests and reminders for Web-based surveys can be done via e-mail with links to the survey embedded in the message.
  - Access and computer literacy is needed for Web-based surveys.
  - Pilot test the survey with people who have different browsers (Archer, 2003; Solomon, 2001).

Interpreting Data

- The nursing professional development educator interprets data from tables, graphs, charts, and so on, and then applies that information to assess learning needs and evaluate outcomes.
  - Bar graph: Displays differences of data characteristics; Y-axis is frequency, X-axis is attributes of the characteristic
  - Histogram: Displays distribution of data; Y-axis is frequency, X-axis is range data, and bars are not separated as they are in a bar graph

- Pareto chart: Displays the relative importance of differences; the left Y-axis is frequency, the right Y-axis is cumulative percentage, and the X-axis lists the attributes of the variable in descending frequency magnitude
- Pie chart: Displays percentages of total for given characteristics
- Control chart: Displays process variation over time; Y-axis is the variable scale, X-axis is time
- Scatter diagram: Displays pairs of data to look for relationship (Polit & Beck, 2007)
- When looking at graphical or tabular data, read the labels or keys to assist with understanding.
- Consider equality of data and environmental circumstances at time of data collection when interpreting.
- Examples of data that the nursing professional development educator interprets are patient, physician, and employee satisfaction; learner characteristics; quality improvement (e.g., handwashing compliance, core measures); course evaluations; and research literature.

Reporting Findings

- Data that the nursing professional development educator reports include budget information, educational activity information, test scores, course evaluations, and performance reviews.
- Qualitative data comes from interviews, focus groups, and open-ended questions on surveys and evaluations.
- The themes of qualitative data are determined from the data and can identify required action, provide descriptions, or support quantitative data.
- Qualitative data is typically reported in narrative form or descriptive tables.
- Quantitative data is numerical and can be reported in tables, charts, and graphs.
- Quantitative data is often aggregated for small group size.
- Reports are given to stakeholders and used for decision-making.

INFORMATION SYSTEMS

Clinical Information Systems

- Hospitals have a variety of information systems:
  - Electronic medical record
  - Admission/discharge/transfer system
  - Order entry
  - Lab reports
  - Radiology reports
  - Pharmacy/medication administration
- Clinical information systems may be fully integrated, partially integrated, or may have no communication between systems.
- Information can be mined from these systems to identify learning needs and/or evaluate learning outcomes.
- The nursing professional development educator needs to identify what data is available and who can assist with access to the information systems.

Educational Information Systems

- Definitions
  - Web server: Software and hardware that sends Web pages to browsers.
  - Web browser: Software that provides the graphical user interface (GUI) of the Internet.
  - Media player: Software that allows audio and video information to be heard and viewed (e.g., Windows Media Player, RealOne Player, Macromedia Flash, QuickTime) via Web browser or computer hardware.
  - Learning management system: Software that coordinates the processes of education and training to include scheduling, registration, billing, launching online courses, and tracking learners' progress and competencies, as well as compiling statistics and reports.
  - Learning content management system: Software for creating, managing, and reusing learning content (e.g., media, pages, tests, course components; Horton & Horton, 2003).
- Learning management systems (LMS) can be purchased from third-party vendors, developed with an organization's resources, or simply be a spreadsheet maintained by the nursing professional development educator.
- Consider what fields can be entered into the LMS (e.g., names and dates of courses, attendees, unit of attendees, test results); these will determine the type of reports the LMS can generate.
- Ensure the process for data entry has minimal measurement error.
- Benefits of LMS include compliance reports for regulatory agencies, validation of competencies, and performance appraisals.
- It is important to identify individual(s) accountable for system maintenance and or updating.

ENVIRONMENTAL SCANNING

- The nursing professional development educator monitors progress, trends, and knowledge in areas of interest to responsibilities.
- Outcomes related to training can be evaluated via quality improvement and risk management (e. g., occurrence/incident reports, core measure data), course evaluations, chart audits, feedback from managers, and staff attrition.
- Use technology to keep current of trends.
  - Web sites
    - Nursing Knowledge International
    - Virginia Henderson International Nursing Library
    - Medscape
    - Nursing Center
    - Specialty organizations
    - Listservs
- Specialty organizations and others offer literature scans in which you select topic areas of interest and receive e-mails with abstracts related to your topic(s).
- Newsletters from specialty organizations and nursing organizations provide timely content.
- Clinical applications are available on personal digital assistants (PDAs) and smartphones.
- Access to a medical library provides availability to current research.

REFERENCES

Archer, T. M. (2003). Web-based surveys. *Journal of Extension, 4*(41). Retrieved from http://www.joe.org/joe/2003august/tt6.php

Bowman, K. R. (2002). Computer skills for educators. In K. L. O'Shea, *Staff development nursing secrets* (pp. 39–46). Philadelphia: Hanley & Belfus.

Horton, W., & Horton, K. (2003). *E-learning tools and technologies.* Indianapolis, IN: Wiley Publishing.

Polit, D. F., & Beck, C. T. (2007). *Nursing research: Generating and assessing evidence for nursing practice.* Philadelphia: Lippincott, Williams & Wilkins.

Solomon, D. J. (2001). Conducting Web-based surveys. *Practical Assessment, Research & Evaluation, 7*(19). Retrieved from http://pareonline.net/getvn.asp?v=7&n=19

24

Contribution to the Nursing Professional Development Specialty

BACKGROUND

- "The nursing professional development educator evaluates his or her own nursing practice in relation to professional practice standards, relevant statues and regulations, and maintenance of continuing professional nursing competence" (American Nurses Association [ANA], 2000, p. 16–17).
- "The nursing professional development educator acquires and maintains current knowledge and competency in nursing professional development practice" (ANA, 2000, p. 17).
- "The nursing professional development educator interacts with, and contributes to the professional development of, peers and other health care providers as colleagues" (ANA, 2000, p. 18).
- The nursing professional development educator contributes to the specialty through role-modeling professional behaviors that are hallmarks of a professional and engaging in professional interactions to support and advance the specialty practice.

Role-Modeling

Certification
- The nursing professional development educator "seeks certification when eligible" (ANA, 2000, p. 17).

- *Certification* recognizes the nurse as having successfully completed an examination in a particular specialty, thereby acknowledging the possession of advanced knowledge.
- Certification of nursing professional development educators provides recognition among peers and in the nursing community for attainment of a specialized body of knowledge (Lewis & Case, 2001).
- Additional reasons for educators to achieve specialty certification in nursing professional development include:
  - Provides an opportunity to affirm knowledge and skills in education
  - Serves as a benchmark for practice
  - Demonstrates ability to function in a nursing professional development role, regardless of practice setting
  - Creates a personal sense of satisfaction and goal attainment (Aucoin, 2002).

Competency

- *Educator competencies* are performance statements that originate from experience, observation, and validation and describe behaviors needed to fulfill educator activities and responsibilities (Wolff, 2002).
- Competencies identified by Wolff (2002)
  - Cognitive domain
    - Applies nursing knowledge and organizational philosophies
    - Demonstrates the educational process (e.g., adult learning principles, needs assessment, program development, educational philosophies)
    - Uses critical thinking skills
  - Psychomotor domain
    - Clinical skills
    - Teaching skills
    - Expert learner skills
    - Physical and motor skills
  - Affective domain
    - Interpersonal skills (e.g., verbal, written, computer)
    - Political savvy
    - Ability to reflect critically about personal characteristics
    - Attitudes, values, and beliefs that complement nursing and teaching roles
    - Professional behaviors
- Competencies identified by Brunt (2007)
  - Designs and revises educational activities
  - Uses a variety of teaching strategies and audiovisuals
  - Uses and evaluates material resources and facilities
  - Conducts needs assessment using a variety of strategies
  - Involves learners in needs assessment and outcomes identification
  - Determines and revises priorities for educational activities
  - Evaluates effectiveness and outcomes of educational endeavors
  - Coordinates complex educational offerings
  - Selects appropriate teaching strategies to facilitate behavioral change
  - Develops curriculums
  - Adjusts content and teaching strategy during presentation based on learners' reactions
  - Creates and applies new educational methodologies

- Uses appropriate measurement methods to assess and document competence
- Possesses expert knowledge of how to teach within organizational culture
- Measures and communicates return on investment

Portfolio

- The nursing professional development educator "maintains a personal portfolio that documents ongoing continuing professional nursing competence" (ANA, 2000, p. 17).
- A portfolio is "material documenting the professional development, career planning, demonstration of learning, and maintenance of continuing professional nursing competence of the individual nurse" (ANA, 2000, p. 25).
- The format of a portfolio can vary but may include these components:
  - Professional credentials
  - Continuing education
  - Leadership activities
  - Narrative self-reflection of practice
  - Documentation of the relevance of professional learning experiences
  - Examples demonstrating competence in a certain area (Brunt, 2007).
- Portfolios can be used to document continuing competence, describe job-related skills and accomplishments, confirm professional development, evaluate performance, and verify that criteria for advancement have been met (Brunt, 2002).
- When building a portfolio:
  - Be selective: include relevant material
  - Be clear and concise: make it easy to read
  - Be coherent: maintain logical flow of content
  - Be professional: use correct grammar and professional style (Brunt, 2007)
- Educators may use these skills to assist others in developing portfolios:
  - Enabling: Supporting individuals while developing a portfolio
  - Educational counseling: Helping individuals explore and understand their learning to develop educational and career goals
  - Advising: Helping individuals interpret information and make decisions
  - Assessing: Assisting individuals to develop confidence in self-assessment to take ownership of their profile
  - Informing: Providing information about learning opportunities and professional development policies (Brunt, 2007)

Professional Self-Development

- Review job expectations and your own knowledge base.
- Find a mentor, either within or outside the organization, to serve as a resource.
- Network with colleagues.
- Identify and act on your own learning needs through ongoing academic or continuing education.
- Attend regional or national meetings in your clinical or education specialty.
- Read journals and books in nursing and related disciplines regularly.
- Set short-term and long-term goals and review goals on a regular basis.
- Participate in activities of professional and specialty organizations (Deck, 2002; Hood, 2002; Lewis & Case, 2001; Sturdivant, 2002).

Professional Interactions

Networking
- Networking with other professionals fosters professional growth.
- Establish networks with other educators within the organization and through involvement in professional organizations locally, regionally, and nationally.
- Electronic mailing forums (e.g., listservs) provide a mechanism to establish a virtual network through which educators can generate discussion or share information about educational topics and trends.
- Networking provides a forum for the exchange of ideas and information to stay current about healthcare issues, clinical developments, educational strategies and trends, and political or regulatory issues that affect the practice of nursing professional development (Lewis & Case, 2001).

Policy Development
- The nursing professional development educator "develops, implements, and evaluates policies and procedures to improve the quality of nursing professional development practice" (ANA, 2000, p. 16).
- Policies provide guidance about specific issues or situations and are a basis for decision-making and action.
- Procedures describe the processes for implementing and operationalizing policies.
- Policies and procedures for nursing professional development may focus on topics such as program development, administration of educational activities, record-keeping, departmental orientation, and resource utilization.
- Policies and procedures must be developed in a collaborative manner and be consistent with departmental and institutional policies and procedures.
- Benefits of policies and procedures:
  - Quick and valid reference to meet employer expectations
  - Method to meet requirements of accrediting and regulatory agencies
  - Consistency and continuity in how certain situations are implemented
  - Facilitate predictable management of situations and activities
  - Minimize the need for repeated decision-making on routine matters (Alspach, 1995)

Mentoring
- Mentoring is a process through which a novice benefits from a relationship with an experienced professional.
- A mentor can guide, direct, counsel, answer questions, provide feedback, and foster networking.
- Mentoring may be formal or informal.
- Nursing professional development educators may serve as mentors to staff nurses and others in the work setting.
- Novice nursing professional development educators benefit from mentoring by experienced educators who can ease anxiety and facilitate integration to the educator role (Lewis & Case, 2001).

Dissemination

- The nursing professional development educator "shares knowledge and skills with colleagues" (ANA, 2000, p. 18).
- Publications
  - Publication is one way to share innovative staff and patient teaching strategies that were successful in addressing educational needs.
  - Writing for publication can be a source of personal satisfaction or professional advancement.
  - When planning to prepare a manuscript for submission, check the journal's "Instructions for Authors" for guidance.
  - Most editors of nursing journals are willing to work with authors to refine a manuscript into acceptable form.
  - The *Journal for Nurses in Staff Development* (JNSD) and the *Journal of Continuing Education in Nursing* (JCEN), as well as other nursing and education journals, are publications to consider for submitting manuscripts about effective educational programs and innovations (Lewis & Case, 2001; Puetz, 2002).
- Presentations
  - Presenting at meetings, conferences, and other professional gatherings is a way to share clinical and educational expertise and experiences with other nursing professional development educators.
  - Presentations may be formal (e.g., keynote speech, concurrent session) or informal (e.g., roundtable discussion, poster).
  - The nature of a presentation depends on several variables:
    - Your abilities and interests
    - Needs and interests of the audience
    - Your goals
    - The nature of the setting (Paterson, 2002)
  - See Chapter 9 for specific information about planning and delivering a presentation.

REFERENCES

Alspach, J. G. (1995). *The educational process in nursing staff development.* St. Louis, MO: Mosby.

American Nurses Association. (2000). *Scope and standards of practice for nursing professional development.* Washington, DC: American Nurses Publishing.

Aucoin, J. W. (2002). Preparing for certification. In B. E. Puetz & J. W. Aucoin (Eds.), *Conversations in nursing professional development* (pp. 375–378). Pensacola, FL: Pohl Publishing.

Brunt, B. A. (2002). Standards of practice. In B. E. Puetz & J. W. Aucoin (Eds.), *Conversations in nursing professional development* (pp. 365–372). Pensacola, FL: Pohl Publishing.

Brunt, B. A. (2007). *Competencies for staff educators: Tools to evaluate and enhance nursing professional development.* Marblehead, MA: HCPro.

Deck, M. L. (2002). Educator. In B. E. Puetz & J. W. Aucoin (Eds.), *Conversations in nursing professional development* (pp. 61–67). Pensacola, FL: Pohl Publishing.

Hood, A. W. (2002). Factors that affect the educator's role. In K. L. O'Shea (Ed.), *Staff development nursing secrets* (pp. 17–25). Philadelphia: Hanley & Belfus.

Lewis, D. J., & Case, B. (2001). The staff development specialist role. In National Nursing Staff Development Organization, *Getting started in clinical and nursing staff development* (2nd ed., pp. 92–98). Pensacola, FL: National Nursing Staff Development Organization.

Paterson, B. L. (2002). Presentation skills. In K. L. O'Shea (Ed.), *Staff development nursing secrets* (pp. 123–129). Philadelphia, PA: Hanley & Belfus.

Puetz, B. E. (2002). Publishing. In B. E. Puetz & J. W. Aucoin (Eds.), *Conversations in nursing professional development* (pp. 391–397). Pensacola, FL: Pohl Publishing.

Sturdivant, M. (2002). Clinical. In B. E. Puetz & J. W. Aucoin (Eds.), *Conversations in nursing professional development* (pp. 103–111). Pensacola, FL: Pohl Publishing.

Wolff, A. C. (2002). Educator competencies. In K. L. O'Shea (Ed.), *Staff development nursing secrets* (pp. 27–37). Philadelphia, PA: Hanley & Belfus.

Review Questions

1. If an NPD educator discusses a learner's performance at a skills lab testing session with colleagues at lunch, which ethical principle is violated?
    a. Autonomy
    b. Beneficence
    c. Confidentiality
    d. Veracity

2. The NPD educator area of responsibility includes 150 employees. The most efficient method for maintaining staff educational records is:
    a. a learning management system.
    b. a printout of an electronic spreadsheet posted on the units.
    c. staff professional portfolios.
    d. unit-based files for employee access for updating.

3. Which evaluation strategy assesses knowledge acquisition?
    a. A pretest and a posttest
    b. Calculation of program expenses compared to profit generated from providing a specific learning activity
    c. Questionnaire pertaining to the learners' perceptions of how well they were able to meet program objectives
    d. Skill return demonstration

4. Commercial support guidelines mandate that:
    a. commercially supplied funds are given in the form of educational grants.
    b. in-kind assistance or funding from a commercial company is acceptable and expected.
    c. presentation of research conducted by a commercial company gives that company the right to influence the design and presentation of any educational activity.
    d. the scientific objectivity of educational activities is subject to the review and approval of the commercial company supporting such activities.

5. The NPD educator is trying to decide which methods and materials to use for a new educational activity. The most important consideration is the:
    a. availability of resources.
    b. length of instruction.
    c. nature of the course objectives.
    d. size of the group.

6. Pausing to ask the learners to evaluate the program halfway through a presentation is an example of what type of evaluation?
    a. Criterion-referenced
    b. Formative
    c. Norm-referenced
    d. Summative

7. An effective tool to demonstrate how the steps of a process are related to each other is a:
    a. cause-and-effect diagram.
    b. flow chart.
    c. histogram.
    d. scatter diagram.

8. Political savvy and the ability to translate ideas into practice are examples of which type of skills used in the consultation process?
    a. Communication skills
    b. Diagnostic skills
    c. Interpersonal skills
    d. Problem-solving skills

9. The NPD educator is working with the staff nurse to develop a plan for career advancement. This is an example of:
    a. coaching.
    b. consulting.
    c. facilitation.
    d. remediation.

10. The purpose of the Institutional Review Board is to:
    a. ensure informed consent is obtained.
    b. ensure research studies follow safety regulations.
    c. protect the institution.
    d. protect research subjects.

11. The first step in establishing an education department is:
    a. communicating the purpose of the department to the staff.
    b. developing objectives that create a climate for learning.
    c. reviewing the goals of the organization.
    d. soliciting ideas from staff who are employed by the organization.

12. Which instructional activity in a program offering on cardiopulmonary resuscitation (CPR) best exemplifies a basic principle of adult education?
    a. Administering a written examination at the end of the CPR course
    b. Evaluating the CPR technique by peers
    c. Explaining how CPR can save lives in the workplace
    d. Reviewing the "ABC's" of CPR

13. A learning objective in the cognitive domain asks the learner to:
    a. correctly remove a colostomy pouch.
    b. demonstrate drawing blood from a central line catheter.
    c. explain personal feelings when caring for patients at the end of life.
    d. identify two risk factors for heart disease.

14. Which teaching strategies best meet the needs of a learner with Kolb's diverger style?
    a. Demonstration and return demonstration using a handout
    b. Group discussion with a follow-up project and report
    c. Lecture supplemented with assigned readings
    d. Self-instruction using computer simulation and games

15. When faced with competing priorities, it is important for the NPD educator to:
    a. consider cost first.
    b. develop personal goals.
    c. plan, organize, and delegate.
    d. set scope limits.

16. The most efficient way to administer an annual needs assessment survey is:
    a. by hand-delivering it to each employee and waiting for them to complete it.
    b. by posting it on a Web site service with a link sent to each employee via e-mail.
    c. to distribute it during staff meetings and collect completed forms at the end of the meetings.
    d. to mail it to each employee's home with a stamped, addressed return envelope.

17. Data sources for identifying learning needs and learning outcomes include:
    a. admission/discharge/transfer data and nurse manager interviews.
    b. course evaluation summaries and number of certified staff.
    c. clinical information systems and incident report trends.
    d. staff satisfaction scores and new grad retention data.

18. Compared to interactive, computer-assisted instruction, the lecture-discussion method of instruction:
    a. allows more content to be covered in a given amount of time.
    b. is less effective in teaching higher-level cognitive concepts.
    c. is more efficient in identifying learning problems.
    d. provides more feedback to learners.

19. The NPD educator is coordinating a seminar for National Nurses Week and has contacted a nationally known speaker to deliver the keynote address. Early in the planning stage, the educator seeks to:
    a. develop a staffing plan with the nurse manager to promote seminar attendance.
    b. generate collaborative agreements with other agencies to increase community participation.
    c. obtain a written agreement from the speaker to confirm honorarium and expense reimbursement.
    d. request copies of the speaker's book from the publisher to use as door prizes at the event.

20. Ongoing competency assessment focuses on:
    a. development of a professional portfolio by registered nurse staff members.
    b. knowledge, skills, and abilities needed during the first 12 months of employment.
    c. new skills and products; changes in practice/equipment; and skills that are high-risk, low-volume, and problem-prone.
    d. practice changes due to policy changes, new equipment, hospital initiatives, and regulatory requirements.

21. To best meet the diverse needs of staff, the NPD educator provides inservices that:
    a. are in the same place and of the same format.
    b. are planned well in advance.
    c. use a consistent format.
    d. use formal and informal learning techniques.

22. The most appropriate method for documenting professional competency is:
    a. 20 hours of continuing education per year.
    b. completion of annual competency checklists.
    c. completion of a professional portfolio.
    d. documented evidence of specialty certification.

23. In demonstrating competence in nursing professional development, the educator's behavior aligns with:
    a. his or her level of graduate education.
    b. hospital and departmental policy and procedures.
    c. the state Nurse Practice Act and ANA Code of Ethics.
    d. content of the specialty certification exam.

24. When selecting faculty for an educational activity, it is important to remember that faculty internal to the organization
    a. are considered to be more "prestigious" than those external to the organization.
    b. are given an honorarium for their services.
    c. understand the organizational values and culture.
    d. usually bring perspectives that are new and different to learning activities.

25. A nursing staff development department that is coordinating a program on back safety plans to post promotional fliers in all nursing conference rooms. To attract the largest audience, the flier includes the program title and which message?
    a. "All nursing personnel, call extension 6338 to register" printed above a map showing the location of the conference room
    b. "All Registered Nurses welcome, 5 p.m., Monday, West Wing Conference Room"
    c. "Refreshments served, presented by Physical Therapy, October 1, 5 p.m."
    d. "West Wing Conference Room, All Nursing Staff, 5 p.m., October 1"

26. The best method for determining what to teach a new nursing employee during orientation involves:
    a. asking the nurse manager for a list of topics to teach the employee.
    b. asking the preceptor what the employee needs to know.
    c. conducting a learning needs assessment with the employee.
    d. following a standard orientation program plan.

27. The NPD educator's cousin is a talented amateur photographer and has taken some wonderful pictures of the buildings and grounds of the healthcare system for which the NPD educator works. The NPD educator is speaking at a national staff development conference and decides to incorporate copies of these pictures as part of the slide presentation. What should the NPD educator do to avoid copyright infringement?
    a. Make copies of the photographs and distribute them as handouts rather than in a slide presentation.
    b. Nothing, because the NPD educator's cousin is not a professional photographer.
    c. Obtain the cousin's permission to use the photographs before incorporating them into the slide presentation.
    d. Use the photographs and tell the cousin that he or she "forgot" to ask permission.

28. Which situation requires educational intervention?
    a. A graduate nurse requests assistance passing the NCLEX-RN.
    b. A nursing assistant is observed failing to follow standard precautions.
    c. A unit nurse educator reports that a newly hired nurse fails to complete electronic documentation.
    d. An oncology staff nurse requests a program on working with families of terminally ill patients.

29. Which statement indicates an accurate assessment of a learning need?
    a. "Nurses on this unit state that they have never worked with unlicensed assistive personnel and need a class on appropriate delegation."
    b. "Our quality review shows 10 medication events this month, indicating a need for a class on medication administration."
    c. "Tuberculosis cases in the state have increased, so we need to hold a learning activity on tuberculosis transmission."
    d. "We have to teach the staff to use the patient care assignment sheets at the beginning of each shift."

30. During a presentation, the NPD educator identifies a lack of interest by the participants. The most appropriate action is to:
    a. ask the audience to share their experiences related to the topic.
    b. continue with the presentation because it is dry, regulatory required content.
    c. give a pop quiz.
    d. give a 10-minute break.

31. Visibility of an electronic slide presentation for a large audience is best when:
    a. graphics are included.
    b. handouts are provided.
    c. the background is lighter than the text.
    d. the font size is at least 24 point.

32. Which is the most important criterion for selecting an educational method?
    a. The method facilitates meeting the learning objectives.
    b. The physical characteristics of the classroom accommodate the method.
    c. The teacher is skillful in, and comfortable with, using the method.
    d. The time allocated for the learning exercise is sufficient.

33. Which situation represents a potential conflict of interest that must be declared at an educational activity?
    a. A conference planning committee member is an expert who has presented on the conference topic
    b. A participant who works for Baxter mentions an infusion product during a small group discussion
    c. A presenter discussing nursing care of the cardiomyopathy patient is a member of Pfizer's speakers' bureau
    d. At a class on ostomy care, the NPD educator has a display table of wound care supplies outside the classroom

34. The most appropriate sources for the NPD educator to use for program outcome effectiveness include:
    a. benchmarking and program evaluation data.
    b. dashboards and posttest scores.
    c. feedback from nurse managers.
    d. quality indicators from Joint Commission.

35. According to cognitive learning theory, learning occurs as a result of:
    a. exposure to positive role models.
    b. information processing and application.
    c. learner insights and the teacher–learner relationship.
    d. repeated practice and reinforcement.

36. When writing behavioral objectives, it is important to remember that:
    a. each objective should contain no more than two expected behaviors.
    b. objectives are developed in terms of what learners must achieve.
    c. programs that deal with abstract concepts do not require measurable objectives.
    d. words such as "understand" and "appreciate" are acceptable due to learning needs.

37. A preceptor complains that the preceptee is "just not getting it." After soliciting an example of the preceptee's behavior from the preceptor, the most appropriate action for the NPD educator is to:
    a. ask the preceptor to join the preceptor support group.
    b. discuss the teaching-learning process with the preceptor.
    c. interview the preceptee.
    d. notify the nurse manager.

38. The NPD educator has been asked to work with a staff member who is having difficulty with ECG interpretation. The most appropriate action for the NPD educator is to:
    a. develop a learning contract with specific dates for completion.
    b. have the staff member retake the ECG course.
    c. listen to the staff member's perspective and mutually set attainable goals.
    d. provide an ECG self-study packet for the staff member to complete.

39. Creating an appropriate climate for change includes:
    a. assuaging employee fear by assuring them that they probably will not lose their jobs.
    b. clearly and honestly relaying both the positive and negative aspects of change.
    c. communicating management's priorities since it is management that will implement the change.
    d. concealing any plans for downsizing because this will only increase resistance to the change.

40. When instituting a quality improvement program for the education department, the most important first action is to:
    a. clearly define the program's purpose and functions and the processes by which services are provided.
    b. design an evaluation program that includes quality control, technology measurement, and performance measurement.
    c. develop an evaluation tool to assess the quality of services provided by the department and the desired outcomes.
    d. implement a quality improvement plan, determine its impact, and document the results.

41. The education department is initiating a quality improvement project related to the inclusion of age-specific care concepts in educational activities. Which data source will provide the most useful data about this indicator?
    a. Chart audits
    b. Educational records
    c. Observation
    d. Test scores

42. In which of the following situations is the educator role modeling professional behaviors?
    a. Asking staff nurses to share information about volunteer experiences in the community
    b. Completing a budget worksheet for a conference planning committee
    c. Participating in a study group to prepare for certification
    d. Using new technology to design an educational activity on palliative care for staff

43. Validity of a test is best demonstrated through the use of:
    a. a test blueprint.
    b. item analysis.
    c. participant feedback.
    d. participant test scores.

44. An action that the NPD educator takes during the "gaining entry" portion of the consultation process is:
    a. completing an environmental scan to identify influencing factors.
    b. conducting a staff survey about barriers to attending educational activities.
    c. developing timelines and goals for achievement during the project.
    d. establishing an action plan for completion of the project.

45. The nurse educator serves as a facilitator by:
    a. creating a formal learning environment using one's own learning style to plan educational activities.
    b. directing team members to their manager if they encounter barriers to success in a project.
    c. having team members complete an evaluation tool to analyze the effectiveness of the team.
    d. volunteering to handle all data collection activities for a problem-solving group.

46. During negotiation, a win-win outcome is best obtained by:
    a. bringing in a neutral party to mediate the issue.
    b. building understanding, support, and acceptance.
    c. compromising and looking for shared interests.
    d. empathetic listening and problem-solving.

47. The majority of management problems result from:
    a. competing priorities.
    b. lack of communication.
    c. organizational complexity.
    d. time pressures.

48. When the unit-based education council becomes unproductive, the nurse manager asks the NPD educator to take over the group. The most appropriate action by the NPD educator is to:
    a. identify problematic feelings and misperceptions among the council members.
    b. provide specific outcomes and timelines for the council members.
    c. realize this is a normal part of team development—storming—that will pass.
    d. show respect to the council members through active listening.

49. Research findings indicate no significant difference in teaching effectiveness when using fact sheets versus lectures. In response, the nurse educator's most appropriate action is to:
    a. continue to use a lecture format because it allows for interaction with the presenter.
    b. discontinue the use of both fact sheet and lecture formats.
    c. make no changes in presentation methods until exploring the findings further.
    d. use both lectures and fact sheets to present information.

50. Due to the nature of educational activities, the majority of research related to professional development education uses what type of research design?
    a. Correlational
    b. Exploratory nonexperimental
    c. Quasi-experimental
    d. Retrospective nonexperimental

Answers to the Review Questions

1. **Correct Answer: C.** The ethical principle of confidentiality refers to the protection of personal information, such as a learner's performance at a skills lab testing session. Autonomy refers to the right of a competent individual to exercise self-determination. Beneficence is the obligation to do good for one's client. Veracity is telling the truth.

2. **Correct Answer: A.** Learning management systems automate record-keeping for job requirements, orientation, ongoing competency, and continuing education. Automation decreases time and error.

3. **Correct Answer: A.** Knowledge acquisition addresses the cognitive learning domain at the second level of evaluation. Tests are the most common measure of the cognitive domain.

4. **Correct Answer: A.** Presentation of research conducted by a commercial company does not give that company the right to influence the design and presentation of any educational activity, nor does the company have the right to evaluate the scientific objectivity of educational activities. In-kind assistance or funding from a commercial company should be acknowledged in printed materials for a learning activity.

5. **Correct Answer: C.** Learning objectives that clearly identify the desired outcomes of the learning process facilitate the selection of teaching strategies and identification of resources needed for successful completion of learning activities.

6. **Correct Answer: B.** Formative evaluation takes place during the learning activity and is used to alter content or teaching methods.

7. **Correct Answer: B.** A flow chart depicts the nature and flow of steps in a process. Cause-and-effect diagrams are pictorial displays that suggest causal relationships of a problem. A histogram is a graphic summary. A scatter diagram is also a graphic representation of data, but is portrayed as an observed relationship between two variables.

8. **Correct Answer: D.** In the consultant role, the NPD educator uses political savvy to accurately analyze the environment when considering possible causes and potential solutions to a problem. The ability to translate ideas into practice allows the consultant to effectively collaborate with clients in designing and implementing problem-solving strategies.

9. **Correct Answer: A.** The NPD educator uses coaching for remediation, career development, and clinical advancement.

10. **Correct Answer: D.** The Institutional Review Board ensures research activities take steps to protect the rights and welfare of humans involved in research.

11. **Correct Answer: C.** The mission, vision, values, and goals of a staff development department must be based on the organizational mission, vision, values, and goals so that educational efforts are consistent with the organizational dynamics.

12. **Correct Answer: C.** Adults need to understand how specific knowledge, skills, and behaviors will benefit them in job performance, interpersonal interactions, and/or professional development. They focus on obtaining knowledge and skills that will help them in their daily lives.

13. **Correct Answer: D.** "Identify" is an action that requires knowledge of facts and therefore is in the cognitive domain. "Remove" and "demonstrate" both relate to the ability to perform psychomotor skills. "Explain feelings" suggests action in the affective domain.

14. **Correct Answer: A.** The learner with a diverger style emphasizes concrete experience and reflective observation (Feeling/Watching). The strategies of demonstration and return demonstration make use of these tendencies as a learner observes then actively performs a skill. Self-instruction, group discussion, and lecture are strategies effective for accommodator, converger, and assimilator styles of learner.

15. **Correct Answer: C.** Prioritization includes planning time and task, organizing activities to facilitate goal achievement, and delegating to make best use of resources.

16. **Correct Answer: B.** Web-based surveys are less costly, provide data easily imported into a form to be uploaded to spreadsheet or statistical software, and can allow for reminders to be linked to those who have not responded. Use of the Web also decreases measurement error introduced by hand data entry and calculation.

17. **Correct Answer: C.** Data from clinical practice records (clinical information systems and incident reports) provide objective information for learning needs assessment. Improvement in data from these sources will reflect the achievement of learning outcomes.

18. **Correct Answer: A.** The lecture-discussion method of instruction is efficient and effective when a large amount of information must be presented to groups. Both methods can be used effectively to teach higher-level cognitive concepts. Lecture is less efficient than computer-assisted instruction in the identification of learning problems and providing learner feedback.

19. **Correct Answer: C.** External presenters require a contract or letter of agreement outlining their needs and expenses. This must be finalized early in the planning process to avoid problems or misunderstandings later. The other planning activities can be done closer to the date of the seminar.

20. **Correct Answer: C.** Ongoing competencies reflect the ever-changing nature of the job that includes not only practice changes but also those practices that are high-risk, low-volume, and problem-prone.

21. **Correct Answer: D.** Inservices need to be flexible to meet learning needs with a variety of teaching styles to accommodate learner preferences.

22. **Correct Answer: C.** The professional portfolio includes demonstration of learning and maintenance of professional competence. Continuing education, checklists, and specialty certification are components of a professional portfolio.

23. **Correct Answer: C.** While competence begins with academic preparation, behaviors of the NPD educator are defined by the nursing scope of practice and code of ethics. Both of these are broader than hospital policy and procedure.

24. **Correct Answer: C.** Faculty from within an organization know the culture, values, and goals of the organization. The other factors identified are more commonly associated with external speakers.

25. **Correct Answer: D.** Information included on the flier includes all the required details that participants need to know to attend the activity—title, location, date, time, and target audience. This will attract the largest audience, as other options require the participant to take action, target a limited audience, or omit key information.

26. **Correct Answer: C.** Learning needs assessment is a systematic process of collecting data that will most accurately identify the new nursing employee's gaps between actual and desired knowledge, skills, and/or attitudes.

27. **Correct Answer: C.** The photographs are the intellectual property of the NPD educator's cousin; therefore, the cousin's permission to use these photographs must be obtained. Other options would be copyright infringement.

28. **Correct Answer: B.** Observation is a needs assessment method that in this situation identifies a gap between actual and desired knowledge, skills, and/or attitudes related to standard precautions. Other choices reflect verbalized requests or suggestions that need further assessment to determine if they are indicators of educational needs or system problems.

29. **Correct Answer: A.** Nursing staff members are an accurate source of needs assessment data when several individuals identify the need and the need is validated by patterns of practice.

30. **Correct Answer: A.** Engaging the audience by introducing their experience with the topic aligns with adult learning principles, thereby enhancing interest.

31. **Correct Answer: D.** A 24-point font ensures text can be read when an electronic slide is projected onto a screen in various room sizes.

32. **Correct Answer: A.** Although the educator considers several criteria in selecting an educational method, the most important criterion is that the method is an effective approach to achieve the learning objectives. Classroom characteristics, time, and teacher skills can all be adapted as necessary.

33. **Correct Answer: C.** Commercial support guidelines identify that any faculty or presenters who have financial relationships with a commercial interest, such as being a member of a speakers' bureau for a pharmaceutical company, must disclose that financial relationship.

34. **Correct Answer: A.** Tools to evaluate program outcome effectiveness reflect the congruence of goals, objectives, and accomplishments. Benchmarking compares accomplishments while program evaluations reflect goals and objectives.

35. **Correct Answer: B.** According to cognitive learning theory, learning is an active process in which the learner uses cognitive skills to reorganize information into new insights and then applies that information. Behavioral learning theory uses repeated practice and reinforcement. Exposure to positive role models is how learning occurs according to social learning theory. Learner insights and the teacher–learner relationship are hallmarks of psychodynamic learning theory.

36. **Correct Answer: B.** Objectives are written in behavioral terms appropriate to the target audience and specifically identify what the learner must achieve in measurable terms.

37. **Correct Answer: B.** During the preceptor experience, the NPD educator supports the preceptor by maintaining contact to guide the teaching-learning process, troubleshoot problems, and monitor the effectiveness and progress of the program.

38. **Correct Answer: C.** When coaching for remediation, analyze the facts; listen to the person's perspective; mutually set realistic and attainable goals; agree on actions to be taken; and follow up to reflect, evaluate, and provide feedback.

39. **Correct Answer: B.** A positive climate for effective change includes communicating information about the change honestly and allowing staff to ask questions and express concerns.

40. **Correct Answer: A.** The first step initiating a quality improvement program is to define the program's purpose and functions and the processes by which services are provided. This information will be used to determine indicators, tools, performance measures, and desired outcomes.

41. **Correct Answer: B.** Educational records include information about themes and content of activities. Chart audits, observation, and test scores provide useful information for other potential quality improvement activities.

42. **Correct Answer: C.** Achieving certification in one's specialty is a professional behavior. Other situations identify aspects that might be part of the NPD educator role.

43. **Correct Answer: A.** Validity demonstrates that the test measures what it was intended to measure. A test blueprint guides content validity by ensuring the questions align with the content and domain level of learning objectives.

44. **Correct Answer: A.** Completion of an environmental scan is an important step in gaining entry before beginning work on the project or problem itself. The other steps follow later in the consultation process.

45. **Correct Answer: C.** The purpose of facilitation is to help others accomplish their goals and keep systems running smoothly. Having team members complete an evaluation tool is one strategy to assess system functions and improve effectiveness if indicated.

46. **Correct Answer: C.** A win-win outcome has both parties being comfortable with the result. Identifying shared interests guides negotiation toward those aspects each party can compromise on while maintaining mutual gains.

47. **Correct Answer: B.** Communicating purpose, reasoning, expectations, and feedback are key to preventing management problems.

48. **Correct Answer: A.** Team-building is enhanced by identifying problematic feelings and misperceptions and then correcting them. These need to be addressed before work can be accomplished.

49. **Correct Answer: C.** The evidence-based practice process involves a search for the best evidence available and a critical review of the evidence before making changes and integrating the evidence into practice.

50. **Correct Answer: B.** In a nonexperimental design, the researcher collects data without introducing an intervention. Exploratory design provides in-depth exploration of a single process or variable. Professional development education typically does not allow the time or environment to introduce an intervention or multiple processes.

Index

cost-effectiveness analysis, 84
credentialing, 49–50
criterion-referenced evaluation, 90
critical path model, 145
cultural diversity, 25
culture, organizational, 11, 12

D
data
 collection methods for, 152–153, 162
 interpretation of, 162–163
 qualitative, 163
 quantitative, 163
data analysis, 153–154
databases, 51, 150
demonstration, 67
dependent variables, 151, 152
direct costs, 84
documentation
 accreditation, 101
 guidelines for, 99–100
dynamics, 11

E
education
 for adult learners, 17, 18, 21–24
 continuing, 45, 58–59
 inservice, 57–58
 learner characteristics, 24–25
 learning theories, 19–21
 mandatory, 45
 principles of adult, 17–18
 for professional development educators, 43–45
educational activities
 budgeting for, 84
 evaluation of, 89–95. *See also* evaluation;
  evaluation data
 facility management for, 85–86
 marketing of, 81–84
 on-site coordination for, 86
 policies related to, 85
 problems related to, 86
 process management for, 85
educational information systems, 164
educational planning
 behavioral objectives, 65
 content determination, 65–66
 evaluation, 69
 faculty and content expert selection, 66
 general principles, 64–65
 implementation, 69
 teaching strategies, 66–69
educational process
 assessment, 62–64
 background, 61–62
e-learning, 77

electronic slides, 75–76
environmental scanning, 164
Erikson, Erik, 9
ethical accountability, 34
ethical issues
 cheating as, 36
 confidentiality as, 36
 conflict of interest as, 35
 plagiarism as, 35–36
 related to consultation, 132
 related to intellectual property, 35. *See also*
  copyright law
ethics, 33
evaluation
 explanation of, 29, 89
 methodologies of, 91–93
 purpose of, 90
 tools of, 93
 types of, 90
evaluation data
 behavior/outcome, 94–95
 function of, 89
 learning/content, 93–94
 reaction/process, 93
 results/impact, 95
 return on investment, 95–96
evidence, 51, 158
evidence-based practice (EBP)
 advantages of, 158
 application of, 159
 barriers to, 158
 explanation of, 157
 steps of, 50, 158
expenditures, 84
Experiential Learning Model (Kolb), 23
experimental research designs, 152
expert opinion, 51
external consultants, 129
external marketing, 81
external validity, 151

F
facilitation
 function of, 135, 136
 situations requiring, 136–137
 skills for, 136
facility management, 85–86
faculty, selection of, 66
FADE model, 145
Family Educational Rights and Privacy Act
 (FERPA), 38
feedback, 108
fiscal management, 122
fishbone diagrams, 126
Five-Stage Change Theory (Rogers), 115
fixed costs, 84

About the Authors

Diane D. DePew, DSN, RN-BC, has dedicated 20 years to nursing education and professional development. She has a BSN from Seton Hall University, New Jersey; a master's from the University of Maryland School of Nursing, with a focus in nursing education; and a doctorate from the University of Alabama at Birmingham School of Nursing. Diane has taught at both the associate and baccalaureate academic levels. She has been a unit-based educator, service line educator, and director of a professional development department. Certified in Nursing Professional Development, Diane developed and provides a certification review course for the American Nurses Credentialing Center exam.

Diane maintains a professional development consulting practice in evaluation, competency, and curriculum design. She is an accomplished item writer, having taught item-writing workshops and contributed to the American Association of Critical-Care Nurses' certification exam. An active member of ANA, NNSDO, and Sigma Theta Tau, Diane shares her knowledge and love of professional development through customized workshops.

Patricia Kummeth, MSN, RN-BC, received her baccalaureate degree from the College of Saint Teresa, Winona, Minnesota, and her master's degree in Adult Health Nursing with a focus in education from the University of Wisconsin-Eau Claire. Much of her nursing career has been spent as a Nursing Education Specialist in the Department of Nursing, Mayo Clinic, Rochester, Minnesota. In that role, she has been responsible for planning, presenting, and evaluating orientation, continuing education, and inservice activities for nurses.

In addition, Patti has served as an appraiser for the American Nurses Credentialing Center Accreditation Program since 1999. She was a member of the ANCC Commission on Accreditation from 1999 to 2002 and the Accreditation Review Committee from 2003 to 2010. She has been certified in Nursing Professional Development through the American Nurses Credentialing Center since 1992 and is currently an ANCC seminar review speaker for that exam.